Advance Praise for
The Behavioral Addictions

"Kudos to Ascher and Levounis for recognizing that addiction is a disease defined symptomatically by the discomfort experienced by an individual in the absence of a particular substrate, and for further recognizing that the substrate may be more than simply a substance that can produce physiologic dependence. The substrate can include emotional states, activities, and pastimes. The addict, to enter recovery, must remain abstinent not merely from dependence-inducing substances, but from all activities that, for that individual, generate a response that ultimately stifles interpersonal relating and intimacy. The editors and their chapter authors recognize this and have taken on the topic in a compelling and constructive manner that will assist the field in moving forward."

Stuart Gitlow, M.D., M.P.H., M.B.A., President, American Society of Addiction Medicine, Chevy Chase, Maryland

"This book raises awareness and fosters understanding of the clinical presentations and approaches to treatment of a new frontier of non-substance addictions, many of which have been engendered by the proliferation and popularization of new technologies. It is a must-have resource for psychiatrists and other behavioral health practitioners."

Annelle B. Primm, M.D., M.P.H., Deputy Medical Director, American Psychiatric Association, Arlington, Virginia

The Behavioral Addictions

The Behavioral Addictions

Edited by

Michael S. Ascher, M.D.
Petros Levounis, M.D., M.A.

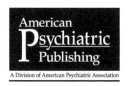

American Psychiatric Publishing
A Division of American Psychiatric Association

Washington, DC
London, England

If you would like to buy between 25 and 99 copies of this or any other American Psychiatric Publishing title, you are eligible for a 20% discount; please contact Customer Service at appi@psych.org or 800–368–5777. If you wish to buy 100 or more copies of the same title, please e-mail us at bulksales@psych.org for a price quote.

Copyright © 2015 American Psychiatric Association
ALL RIGHTS RESERVED

Manufactured in the United States of America on acid-free paper
18 17 16 15 14   5 4 3 2 1
First Edition

Typeset in Minion Pro and Trade Gothic LT

American Psychiatric Publishing
A Division of American Psychiatric Association
1000 Wilson Boulevard
Arlington, VA 22209–3901
www.appi.org

Library of Congress Cataloging-in-Publication Data

Behavioral addictions (Ascher)
  The behavioral addictions / edited by Michael S. Ascher, Petros Levounis.—First edition.
      p. ; cm.
  Includes bibliographical references and index.
  ISBN 978-1-58562-485-0 (pbk. : alk. paper)
  I. Ascher, Michael S., 1980– , editor. II. Levounis, Petros, editor. III. American Psychiatric Association, issuing body. IV. Title.
  [DNLM: 1. Behavior, Addictive—therapy. WM 176]
  RC552.R44
  616.86—dc23
                                                                              2014035470

British Library Cataloguing in Publication Data
A CIP record is available from the British Library.

Contents

Part I. Introduction

Part II. The Behavioral Addictions

Contributors

Michael S. Ascher, M.D.
Clinical Associate in Psychiatry, University of Pennsylvania, Perelman School of Medicine, Philadelphia, Pennsylvania

Jonathan Avery, M.D.
Assistant Professor of Psychiatry, Weill Cornell Medical College, New York, New York

Timothy K. Brennan, M.D.
Associate Director, Fellowship in Addiction Medicine, The Addiction Institute of New York; Clinical Instructor of Pediatrics, Weill Cornell Medical College, New York, New York

Alexis Briggie, Ph.D.
Staff Psychologist, Center for Motivation and Change, New York, New York

Clifford Briggie, Psy.D., LADC, LCSW
Senior Clinician and On-Site Behavioral Health Director, Community Health Center, Meriden, Connecticut

Lisa J. Cohen, Ph.D.
Professor of Psychiatry, Department of Psychiatry, Mount Sinai Beth Israel, New York, New York

Elias Dakwar, M.D.
Assistant Professor, Department of Psychiatry, Columbia University, New York, New York

Emily Deringer, M.D.
Addiction Fellow, Department of Psychiatry, New York University School of Medicine, New York, New York

Eric Y. Drogin, J.D., Ph.D., ABPP
Clinical Instructor, Department of Psychiatry, Harvard Medical School; Member, Program in Psychiatry and the Law, Beth Israel Deaconess Medical Center, Boston, Massachusetts

Jessica A. Gold, M.D., M.S.
Psychiatry Resident, Stanford University School of Medicine, Palo Alto, California

Mark S. Gold, M.D.
Psychiatry Chairman, Dizney Eminent Scholar, and UF Alumni Distinguished Professor, University of Florida, College of Medicine, Gainesville, Florida

Nicole Guanci, M.D.
Chief Resident, Department of Psychiatry, Rutgers New Jersey Medical School, Newark, New Jersey

Yu-Heng Guo, M.D.
Chief Resident of Psychiatry, Department of Psychiatry, Hospital of the University of Pennsylvania; Philadelphia VA Medical Center, Philadelphia, Pennsylvania

Samson Gurmu, M.D.
Director, Women's Unit, Ann Klein Forensic Center, Division of Mental Health Services, West Trenton, New Jersey

Carolyn J. Heckman, Ph.D.
Associate Professor, Cancer Prevention and Control Program, Fox Chase Cancer Center, Philadelphia, Pennsylvania

Yael Holoshitz, M.D.
Clinical Fellow in Public Psychiatry, New York State Psychiatric Institute/New York Presbyterian-Columbia University Medical Center, New York, New York

Najeeb Hussain, M.D.
Assistant Professor, Department of Psychiatry, Rutgers New Jersey Medical School, Newark, New Jersey

Daniel Lache, M.D.
Addictions Fellow, Philadelphia VA Medical Center, University of Pennsylvania Perelman School of Medicine, Philadelphia, Pennsylvania

Petros Levounis, M.D., M.A.
Chair, Department of Psychiatry, Rutgers New Jersey Medical School, Newark, New Jersey; Chief of Service, University Hospital, Newark, New Jersey

Sean X. Luo, M.D., Ph.D.
Leon Levy Fellow in Translational Neuroscience, Department of Psychiatry, Columbia University; The New York State Psychiatric Institute, New York, New York

Omar Mohamed, B.A.
Medical Student, Rutgers New Jersey Medical School, Newark, New Jersey

Sabina Mushtaq, M.D.
Assistant Professor, Director, and Training Director, Division of Child and Adolescent Psychiatry, Department of Psychiatry, Rutgers New Jersey Medical School, New Brunswick, New Jersey

Dmitry Ostrovsky, B.A.
Senior Medical Student, Rutgers New Jersey Medical School, Newark, New Jersey

Nancy M. Petry, Ph.D.
Professor, University of Connecticut Health Center, Calhoun Cardiology Center—Behavioral Health, Farmington, Connecticut

Marc N. Potenza, M.D., Ph.D.
Director, Yale Center of Excellence in Gambling Research, Director, Women and Addictions Core of Women's Health Research at Yale, and Professor of Psychiatry, Child Study and Neurobiology, Yale University School of Medicine, New Haven, Connecticut

Carla J. Rash, Ph.D.
Assistant Professor, University of Connecticut Health Center, Calhoun Cardiology Center—Behavioral Health, Farmington, Connecticut

Mahreen Raza, M.D.
Chief Resident, Department of Psychiatry, Rutgers New Jersey Medical School, Newark, New Jersey

Robert L. Sadoff, M.D.
Clinical Professor of Forensic Psychiatry, and Director, Division of Forensic Psychiatry, and Director, Forensic Psychiatry Fellowship Program, Perelman School of Medicine, University of Pennsylvania, Philadelphia, Pennsylvania

Tolga Taneli, M.D.
Assistant Professor, Director, and Training Director, Division of Child and Adolescent Psychiatry, Department of Psychiatry, Rutgers New Jersey Medical School, New Brunswick, New Jersey

Kimberly A. Teitelbaum, ARNP
Board Certified Psychiatry/Mental Health and Adult Nurse Practitioner, Department of Psychiatry, University of Florida, College of Medicine, Gainesville, Florida

Justine Wittenauer, M.D.
Child and Adolescent Psychiatry Fellow, Department of Psychiatry, Cambridge Health Alliance/Harvard Medical School, Cambridge, Massachusetts

Tauheed Zaman, M.D.
Addiction Psychiatry Fellow, University of California San Francisco, San Francisco, California

Erin Zerbo, M.D.
Assistant Professor, Department of Psychiatry, Rutgers New Jersey Medical School, Newark, New Jersey

Disclosure of Competing Interests

The following contributor to this book has indicated a financial interest in or other affiliation with a commercial supporter, a manufacturer of a commercial product, a provider of a commercial service, a nongovernmental organization, and/or a government agency, as listed below:

Mark S. Gold, M.D.—*Board of Directors:* Axogen, Xhale, HyGreen, Viewray. None of these companies are related to the content of the chapter.

The following contributors to this book have indicated no competing interests to disclose during the year preceding manuscript submission:

Michael S. Ascher, M.D.

Jonathan Avery, M.D.

Timothy K. Brennan, M.D.

Alexis Briggie, Ph.D.

Clifford Briggie, Psy.D., LADC, LCSW

Lisa J. Cohen, Ph.D.

Elias Dakwar, M.D.

Emily Deringer, M.D.

Eric Y. Drogin, J.D., Ph.D., ABPP

Jessica A. Gold, M.D., M.S.

Nicole Guanci, M.D.

Yu-Heng Guo, M.D.

Samson Gurmu, M.D.

Carolyn J. Heckman, Ph.D.

Yael Holoshitz, M.D.

Najeeb Hussain, M.D.

Daniel Lache, M.D.

Petros Levounis, M.D., M.A.

Sean X. Luo, M.D., Ph.D.

Sabina Mushtaq, M.D.

Dmitry Ostrovsky, B.A.

Nancy M. Petry, Ph.D.

Carla J. Rash, Ph.D.

Mahreen Raza, M.D.

Robert L. Sadoff, M.D.

Tolga Taneli, M.D.

Kimberly A. Teitelbaum, ARNP

Justine Wittenauer, M.D.

Tauheed Zaman, M.D.

Erin Zerbo, M.D.

Preface

WE are often asked if behavioral addictions, such as shopping, food, sex, love, texting, e-mailing, and gambling, are really bona fide medical conditions or just an exaggeration of everyday social and personal ailments.

While there is little doubt that these conditions provide unique and poorly researched challenges in everyday clinical practice, the overarching hallmarks of addiction—continued engagement in an action despite negative consequences and loss of control over one's own life—seem to be quite similar for both substances and behaviors that hijack a person's pleasure and reward brain circuitry.

Furthermore, extreme forms of behavioral addictions share a number of specific characteristics with the severe forms of substance use disorders. Four major symptoms can be readily recognized in most addictions, whether they are substance driven, like cocaine and tobacco use disorders, or simply behaviorally driven, like gambling and shopping:

1. The need to use the substance or perform the troublesome behavior at higher doses, or more and more frequently, in order to achieve the same effect—*tolerance* in medical terminology
2. The uncomfortable feeling of being restless, irritable, and discontent, or a flat-out devastating condition, following abrupt discontinuation of the substance or the behavior—*withdrawal* in medical terminology
3. An obsession that seems to "eat" the person from within—in other words, having little interest in anything other than the addictive agent—constantly coming back to "How am I going to use?" "How am I going to pay for it?" "How am I going to come down?" "How am I going to start the process all over again?"
4. External consequences of the addiction in terms of the person's finances, health, interpersonal relationships, legal affairs, etc.

The Diagnostic and Statistical Manual (DSM) system of the American Psychiatric Association continues to be a work in progress, and whereas gambling disorder falls under the "Substance-Related and Addictive Disorders" chapter of DSM-5 (American Psychiatric Association 2013), Internet gaming disorder is subsumed under Section III, the section of DSM-5 reserved for conditions that require further research. The remainder of the behavioral addictions are either not included in DSM-5 or fall under the "Disruptive, Impulse-Control, and Conduct Disorder" chapter.

With this book, we hope to provide a way for clinicians to understand and organize conditions that may not be clearly delineated in DSM-5. The first two chapters of this volume provide an overview of the behavioral addictions from neurobiological, theoretical, clinical, and forensic perspectives. Following this introduction, we present 12 case studies on exercise, food, gambling, Internet gaming, Internet surfing, e-mailing and texting, kleptomania, sex, love, shopping, tanning, and work.

Through the study of real-life cases, we set out to help both trainees and practicing clinicians alike to digest the currently available research and gain some "hands-on" experience with the current diagnosis and treatment of these conditions. Readers can solidify their knowledge by 1) reviewing key points, 2) answering multiple-choice questions at the end of each chapter, and 3) viewing representative scenes from the accompanying videos. Our goal is to create a volume that is informative, practical, and fun!

When it comes to the behavioral addictions, we have a lot more work to do: figuring out reliable diagnostic criteria, building useful assessment tools, and developing effective psychosocial and pharmacological treatments, to name a few critical tasks. We are deeply indebted to our colleagues at the University of Pennsylvania, Rutgers New Jersey Medical School, and many other academic institutions around the United States and abroad for their brilliant contributions to this line of scholarship. We also would like to thank our wonderful filmmakers: Henry B. Lee, Pak Kei Cheung, and Lukas Hassel, who shot the accompanying videos for the book, and our amazingly talented actors most of whom double as medical students at Rutgers New Jersey Medical School: Annica Tehim, Charles Kreisel, Erin Zerbo, Harry Hurley, Jessica Goldman, Jordana Goldman, Ketan Hirapara, Khushboo Baldev, Matthew Sumicad, Nahil Chohan, Omar Mohamed, and Ragha Suresh. Asha Martin and Dmitry Ostrovsky organized the troops and showed great leadership as presidents of PsychSIGN, the Psychiatry medical student interest group at Rutgers. We are grateful for the diligent and attentive work of the American Psychiatric Publishing team.

Finally, a very special acknowledgment goes out to our spouses Lauren Ascher and Lukas Hassel, who, right now, are exhaling a sigh of relief as our little labor of love is going to print. Thank you, Lauren and Lukas, for your tireless dedication, support, and love—and we promise: no more books for another month or two…

Michael Ascher, M.D.
Petros Levounis, M.D., M.A.
October 2014

Reference

American Psychiatric Association: Diagnostic and Statistical Manual of Mental Disorders, 5th Edition. Arlington, VA, American Psychiatric Association, 2013

Video Guide

The Video Learning Experience

The companion videos can be viewed online at **www.appi.org/Ascher**.

Each of the six video vignettes sets out to briefly capture a clinical encounter in which patient and clinician are exploring different behavioral addictions. When viewed in tandem with reading of the book, these six short videos provide a visual and audial learning experience.

Using the Book and the Videos Together

We recommend that readers use the boldface video prompts ▶ embedded in the text as signals for viewing the associated clips in the online viewer at www.appi.org/Ascher. The cues identify the vignettes by title and run time. (The videos are optimized for most current operating systems, including mobile operating systems iOS 5.1 and Android 4.1 and higher.) Chapters 4, 5, 6, 9, 10, and 11 have associated videos.

Description of the Videos

Each of the six videos presents a brief patient interview.

Chapter 4: Diagnosing food addiction (7:06)

The video portrays role modeling of the clinical encounter between the patient and her therapist. Note how the therapist elicits the different criteria for diagnosis of food addiction according to the Yale Food Addiction Scale. Be sure to pay particular attention to the relationship between food and mood for the patient and the role food plays in her current and past life.

Chapter 5: Introductory therapist-patient exchange (6:00)

This vignette is an enactment of the introductory exchange between patient and therapist. Note the role "chasing his losses" (a diagnostic criteria) plays in the patient's gambling pattern and related consequences. The patient mentions gambling as a strategy to make money and rectify his finances; this idea will be a major trigger for gambling urges during the early phase of treatment.

Chapter 6: Establishing rapport and assessing for Internet gaming disorder (4:46)

This video presents a typical encounter with a patient with Internet gaming disorder. Note how the doctor establishes rapport with the patient by asking what specific games he plays and using lingo such as "avatar." Pay close attention to how the doctor elicits the criteria for Internet gaming disorder during the encounter. Also, note how the doctor does a good job of screening for other associated behavioral addictions that are correlated with the Internet, such as gambling and sex addictions.

Chapter 9: Kleptomania: getting the history (5:57)

This video clinical encounter demonstrates how the therapist remains neutral yet persistent in her attempts to help the patient open up about her shoplifting. Given the highly secretive nature of the disorder, patients are often reluctant to talk about the behavior at all. Clinicians should consider asking about it routinely during initial evaluations to indicate that they are familiar with the behavior.

Chapter 10: Addressing motivation to change in sexual addiction (5:23)

This dramatization is a therapy session with a patient suffering from sex addiction. Notice how the patient alternates between seeing his sexual behavior as problematic and as personally acceptable. Notice also the personal meaning the behavior has for this particular patient: the sexual behavior serves a self-soothing function in the context of perceived abandonment. Whereas compulsive sexual behavior may be quite similar across different patients, the personal meaning ascribed to it may be unique to the patient's life history.

Chapter 11: Power of therapeutic alliance (6:20)

The video depicts a clinical encounter, exemplifying how the here-and-now relationship between patient and therapist can be used to facilitate insight into the patient's relationships with others. In the treatment of love addiction, as the therapeutic alliance deepens, the relationship can be an incredibly powerful therapeutic tool to promote insight and effect change.

Video Credits

We thank our wonderful filmmakers Pak Kei Cheung, Lukas Hassel, and Henry B. Lee who shot the accompanying videos for the book and our amazingly talented volunteer actors and organizers: Khushboo Baldev, Nahil Chohan, Jessica Goldman, Jordana Goldman, Ketan Hirapara, Harry Hurley, Charles Kreisel, Asha Martin, Omar Mohamed, Dmitry Ostrovsky, Matthew Sumicad, Ragha Suresh, Annica Tehim, and Erin Zerbo.

Note. The clinical cases portrayed are fictional. Any resemblance to real persons is purely coincidental. The videos feature the work of volunteer clinicians and actor patients who agreed to demonstrate commonly used interview techniques.

PART I

INTRODUCTION

CHAPTER 1

Helping People Behave Themselves

Identifying and Treating Behavioral Addictions

Marc N. Potenza, M.D., Ph.D.

SUBSTANCE addictions currently represent some of the costliest conditions for society, and they often exert tremendous negative impacts on the addicted individuals and those close to them (Uhl and Grow 2004). However, the total cost and impact of addictions may not be entirely captured by data, particularly given debates regarding the boundaries of addiction. These debates, which occur in lay and academic communities, include discussions regarding where to draw the line between healthy and unhealthy levels of participation (Cloud 2012), as well as which behaviors might be considered addictions (Avena et al. 2012; Ziauddeen et al. 2012).

For decades, there has been debate regarding the definition and use of the term addiction. The word *addiction* is derived from Latin, and in its original usage, it connoted being bound to or enslaved by something—although this something was not alcohol or drugs (Maddux and Desmond 2000). Over time, the word became linked to excessive and interfering patterns of alcohol use and then excessive and interfering patterns of drug use, so that by the 1980s, expert consensus was that addiction may be defined as compulsive drug use (O'Brien et al. 2006). Despite this consensus, the term addiction was not included in 1980, 1987, and 1994 in the *Diagnostic and Statistical Manual of Mental Disorders* (DSM-III, DSM-III-R, and DSM-IV [American Psychiatric Association 1980,

1987, 1994]), and the diagnostic terms of substance abuse and dependence were used in definitions of substance use disorders.

Around this time, questions also existed about the extent to which non-substance-related conditions might share features with substance use disorders and be considered addictions (Holden 2001; Potenza et al. 2001; Shaffer 1999), although suggestions of similarities between specific non-substance and substance behaviors were identified previously. For example, Gamblers Anonymous, whose tenets are based on those of Alcoholics Anonymous, was founded in 1957, and criteria for pathological gambling, the diagnostic entity introduced in 1980 into DSM-III, show similarities with those for substance dependence, including criteria assessing tolerance, withdrawal, interference in major areas of life functioning, and repeated unsuccessful attempts to cut back or quit. These similarities are also echoed in proposed core elements of addiction: 1) continued engagement in a behavior despite adverse consequences, 2) an appetitive urge or craving state prior to engagement in the behavior, 3) compulsive engagement in the behavior, and 4) diminished or lost control (Shaffer 1999). Despite these similarities, pathological gambling was classified in DSM-III, DSM-III-R, and DSM-IV as an impulse-control disorder "Not Elsewhere Classified," separate from substance use disorders.

Research work groups convened in preparation for DSM-5 considered data relevant to the classification of pathological gambling and other non-substance-related conditions, reviewing materials relevant to their consideration as non-substance or behavioral addictions or as impulsive-compulsive-spectrum disorders (Petry 2006; Potenza 2006; Potenza et al. 2009). These summaries and other data were used by DSM-5 committees to consider the most appropriate definitions and classifications of pathological gambling and other impulse-control disorders, and this work led to the reclassification of pathological gambling (now termed gambling disorder) as a behavioral addiction in DSM-5 (American Psychiatric Association 2013; Holden 2010; Petry et al. 2013). This reclassification of gambling disorder as the first (and currently only) behavioral addiction in DSM-5 lends credence to the construct of behavioral addictions and provides precedent for the future consideration of other behavioral addictions in future editions of DSM.

Behavioral addictions in other (nongambling) domains have been proposed, and some were considered in the preparation of DSM-5. For example, the committee considering substance-related and addictive disorders also considered problematic Internet use and problematic video game playing (conditions that have been called Internet addiction or gaming addiction, respectively), introducing criteria for Internet gaming disorder into Section III ("Emerging Measures and Models") of DSM-5—the section for disorders needing additional study (Petry and O'Brien 2013). Additionally, other committees considered other disorders that may be considered addictive in nature; for example, hypersexual disorder, a condition that some have termed sexual addiction, was considered but not included in DSM-5 (Kor et al. 2013; Reid 2013; Reid et al. 2012). Importantly, for some of these conditions, the committees believed that there were insufficient data at the time to introduce formal diagnoses into DSM-5, highlighting the need for additional research on these conditions.

As clinicians, we are faced with helping people with their ailments with the knowledge that we have available. While reviews are available summarizing current clinical, phenomenological, genetic, and neurobiological data on behavioral addictions (Grant et al. 2013; Leeman and Potenza 2013), few existing sources provide case-based references to help guide clinicians in this rapidly changing area. Thus, *The Behavioral Addictions* represents an important resource for clinicians. *The Behavioral Addictions* covers multiple conditions that represent important clinical entities, including gambling and Internet-related behaviors. Given the recent increase in the availability and use of digital technologies and the problems that people may encounter when using these technologies to excess (Walsh et al. 2013; Yau et al. 2012), *The Behavioral Addictions* includes three chapters related to technological addictions: 1) e-mailing and texting, 2) Internet gaming, and 3) Internet surfing. DSM-5 has grouped gaming and Internet use together as Internet gaming disorder (American Psychiatric Association 2013; Petry and O'Brien 2013; Petry et al., 2014). Some individuals may use the Internet problematically in nongaming fashions, and thus this book recognizes and addresses these topics in separate chapters. This approach seems clinically important because problematic use of technologies for different reasons may affect different groups to varying extents and with varying consequences; for example, use of digital technologies while driving may be particularly hazardous for teenagers who are novice drivers (Klauer et al. 2014).

Other areas covered include sex and romance, domains that may be theoretically linked but may also represent distinct clinical constructs (Frascella et al. 2010; Kor et al. 2013). For example, individuals who engage addictively in sex may represent a different clinical group with distinct needs from those individuals who are consumed by romance. Although kleptomania was not reclassified as a behavioral addiction in DSM-5 and criteria for compulsive shopping or buying were not included in DSM-5, these conditions have been considered behavioral addictions and are also covered in *The Behavioral Addictions* (Black 2013; Grant et al. 2013). Additional topics covered include exercise, tanning, and work, domains that have been cited as addictive for some individuals (Holden 2001; Lichtenstein et al. 2014; Petit et al. 2014). Finally, there is a chapter focusing on food addiction. Although there is currently debate regarding the extent to which food addiction exists, there are multiple similarities between addictive patterns of eating and drug use, with perhaps the group of individuals with binge-eating disorder most likely to display features of food addiction (Gearhardt et al. 2011a). Given the rising estimates of the prevalence of obesity in the past several decades and the changes in the availability of and access to palatable, highly caloric foods, there exist significant public health and clinical implications for considering food within an addiction framework (Gearhardt et al. 2011b).

Taken together, the chapters in *The Behavioral Addictions* represent an important resource for clinicians. As additional information becomes available on these conditions, it can be incorporated into the clinical foundation that these cases provide for readers.

References

American Psychiatric Association: Diagnostic and Statistical Manual of Mental Disorders, 3rd Edition. Washington, DC, American Psychiatric Association, 1980

American Psychiatric Association: Diagnostic and Statistical Manual of Mental Disorders, 3rd Edition, Revised. Washington, DC, American Psychiatric Association, 1987

American Psychiatric Association: Diagnostic and Statistical Manual of Mental Disorders, 4th Edition. Washington, DC, American Psychiatric Association, 1994

American Psychiatric Association: Diagnostic and Statistical Manual of Mental Disorders, 5th Edition. Arlington, VA, American Psychiatric Association, 2013

Avena NM, Gearhardt AN, Gold MS, et al: Tossing the baby out with the bathwater after a brief rinse? The potential downside of dismissing food addiction based on limited data. Nat Rev Neurosci 13(7):514, author reply 514, 2012 22714023

Black DW: Behavioural addictions as a way to classify behaviours. Can J Psychiatry 58(5):249–251, 2013 23756284

Cloud J: What counts as crazy? Time March 19, 2012. Available at: http://content.time.com/time/magazine/article/0,9171,2108584,00.html. Accessed March 15, 2014.

Frascella J, Potenza MN, Brown LL, et al: Shared brain vulnerabilities open the way for nonsubstance addictions: carving addiction at a new joint? Ann N Y Acad Sci 1187:294–315, 2010 20201859

Gearhardt AN, White MA, Potenza MN: Binge eating disorder and food addiction. Curr Drug Abuse Rev 4(3):201–207, 2011a 21999695

Gearhardt AN, Grilo CM, DiLeone RJ, et al: Can food be addictive? Public health and policy implications. Addiction 106(7):1208–1212, 2011b 21635588

Grant JE, Schreiber LR, Odlaug BL: Phenomenology and treatment of behavioural addictions. Can J Psychiatry 58(5):252–259, 2013 23756285

Holden C: 'Behavioral' addictions: do they exist? Science 294(5544):980–982, 2001 11691967

Holden C: Behavioral addictions debut in proposed DSM-V. Science 327(5968):935, 2010 20167757

Klauer SG, Guo F, Simons-Morton BG, et al: Distracted driving and risk of road crashes among novice and experienced drivers. N Engl J Med 370(1):54–59, 2014 24382065

Kor A, Fogel Y, Reid RC, et al: Should hypersexual disorder be classified as an addiction? Sex Addict Compulsivity 20(1–2):27–47, 2013 24273404

Leeman RF, Potenza MN: A targeted review of the neurobiology and genetics of behavioural addictions: an emerging area of research. Can J Psychiatry 58(5):260–273, 2013 23756286

Lichtenstein MB, Christiansen E, Elklit A, et al: Exercise addiction: a study of eating disorder symptoms, quality of life, personality traits and attachment styles. Psychiatry Res 215(2):410–416, 2014 24342179

Maddux JF, Desmond DP: Addiction or dependence? Addiction 95(5):661–665, 2000 10885040

O'Brien CP, Volkow N, Li TK: What's in a word? Addiction versus dependence in DSM-V. Am J Psychiatry 163(5):764–765, 2006 16648309

Petit A, Lejoyeux M, Reynaud M, et al: Excessive indoor tanning as a behavioral addiction: a literature review. Curr Pharm Des 20(25):4070–4075(6), 2014 24001299

Petry NM: Should the scope of addictive behaviors be broadened to include pathological gambling? Addiction 101(Suppl 1):152–160, 2006 16930172

Petry NM, O'Brien CP: Internet gaming disorder and the DSM-5. Addiction 108(7):1186–1187, 2013 23668389

Petry NM, Blanco C, Stinchfield R, et al: An empirical evaluation of proposed changes for gambling diagnosis in the DSM-5. Addiction 108(3):575–581, 2013 22994319

Petry NM, Rehbein F, Gentile DA, et al: An international consensus for assessing Internet gaming disorder using the new DSM-5 approach. Addiction 109(9):1399–1406, 2014 24456155

Potenza MN: Should addictive disorders include non-substance-related conditions? Addiction 101(suppl 1):142–151, 2006 16930171

Potenza MN, Kosten TR, Rounsaville BJ: Pathological gambling. JAMA 286(2):141–144, 2001 11448261

Potenza MN, Koran LM, Pallanti S: The relationship between impulse-control disorders and obsessive-compulsive disorder: a current understanding and future research directions. Psychiatry Res 170(1):22–31, 2009 19811840

Reid RC: Personal perspectives on hypersexual disorder. Sex Addict Compulsivity 20:4–18, 2013

Reid RC, Carpenter BN, Hook JN, et al: Report of findings in a DSM-5 field trial for hypersexual disorder. J Sex Med 9(11):2868–2877, 2012 23035810

Shaffer HJ: Strange bedfellows: a critical view of pathological gambling and addiction. Addiction 94(10):1445–1448, 1999 10790897

Uhl GR, Grow RW: The burden of complex genetics in brain disorders. Arch Gen Psychiatry 61(3):223–229, 2004 14993109

Walsh JL, Fielder RL, Carey KB, et al: Female college students' media use and academic outcomes: results from a longitudinal cohort study. Emerg Adulthood 1(3):219–232, 2013 24505554

Yau YHC, Crowley MJ, Mayes LC, et al: Are Internet use and video-game-playing addictive behaviors? Biological, clinical and public health implications for youths and adults. Minerva Psichiatr 53(3):153–170, 2012 24288435

Ziauddeen H, Farooqi IS, Fletcher PC: Obesity and the brain: how convincing is the addiction model? Nat Rev Neurosci 13(4):279–286, 2012 22414944

CHAPTER 2

Forensic Implications of Behavioral Addictions

Robert L. Sadoff, M.D.
Eric Y. Drogin, J.D., Ph.D., ABPP
Samson Gurmu, M.D.

ADDICTIVE disorders may be divided into two general classifications:

1. Substance-related addictions (alcohol, drugs, medications, tobacco, other substances)
2. Non-substance-related addictions, otherwise known as behavioral addictions (including pathological gambling, kleptomania, pyromania, compulsive buying, compulsive sexual behavior, compulsive exercising, workaholism, Internet addiction)

In the second group, we may separate the behavioral addictions into two major groups:

1. Those that have forensic implications (gambling, Internet gaming, Internet addiction, kleptomania, sexual addiction, buying addiction, pyromania)
2. Those without obvious forensic implications (compulsive exercising, compulsive eating, compulsive tanning, other physical compulsive behaviors including hair pulling [trichotillomania] and excoriation [skin pulling])

Although not with any obvious forensic implication, individuals who fall into the second group may also have issues with the law if their compulsions interfere with work and they get fired for missing time at work or for utilizing work time to carry out their compulsive behaviors. These individuals might sue for discrimination or make a case for having what they consider to be a legitimate medical or mental disorder that requires accommodation and treatment.

In this chapter, we are concerned only with those behavioral addictions that have obvious forensic implications of criminal, civil, or administrative legal difficulties.

It is generally accepted that behavioral disorders, including behavioral addictions, are those that cause the individual anxiety; personal difficulties; depression; or social, familial, or legal problems. Clearly, any excessive behavior could cause intrapersonal disorder and often interpersonal problems. However, some will not lead to legal or forensic difficulties, such as food addiction (unless the food is stolen), compulsive exercising, or workaholism. Clearly, gambling addiction, Internet addiction, sexual addiction, kleptomania, pyromania, and other forms of obsessive-compulsive behavior that cross the social/legal boundaries can lead to forensic difficulties for the individual.

Background

It is well known that a significant percentage of prisoners have both mental and addictive problems (primarily substance abuse) that have affected their judgment, impulse control, and behavior and that cause the individual to commit criminal behaviors that lead to incarceration. However, it is less clear whether the non-substance addictions or the behavioral addictions have similar chemical substrates that affect a person's free will or voluntary behavior.

The word addiction derives from the Latin root *addictus,* a legal term referring to "the lesser person enslaved for debt or theft." As such, *addiction* captures the loss of personal control experienced by people we identify as addicts. However, this perceived loss of control, which is considered the core feature of addiction, has traditionally been codified into diagnostic entities only for drugs and alcohol (Grant et al. 2010). It is now recognized that a wide variety of repetitive behaviors such as gambling, sex, shopping, Internet use, video game playing, and stealing could acquire an irresistible quality and wreak havoc on the lives of the afflicted (Black 2013). But are they truly addictions?

A related concern is which behaviors are categorized as behavioral addictions and which are not? A recent editorial noted that even the foremost experts do not agree on what particular disorders qualify as behavioral addictions (Black 2013). Broadly speaking, behavioral addictions are characterized by behaviors that produce short-term reward and engender persistent behavior despite the knowledge of adverse consequences (Grant et al. 2013). These behaviors include pathological gambling, compulsive sexual behavior, compulsive buying, compulsive Internet use or Internet addiction, compulsive video game playing, binge-eating disorder, kleptomania, and pyromania (Black 2013). While the compulsive quality these behaviors can achieve is largely agreed upon, the nosological status of most of the preceding disordered behaviors is far from certain (Frascella et al. 2010). DSM-5 (American Psychiatric Association 2013) recognizes gambling disorder only under "Substance-Related and Addictive Disorders."

A practical way of addressing the issue of whether out-of-control pleasurable behaviors constitute an addictive process akin to substance addiction is to look at similarities and differences between the two in terms of phenomenology, natural history, comorbidity, genetics, and putative neurobiological mechanisms (Grant et al. 2010).

The natural history of many of the behavioral addictions is similar to that of substance addiction (Grant et al. 2013). Both share a similar onset age: adolescence and young adulthood (Chambers and Potenza 2003). Behavioral addictions, like substance use disorders, exhibit a chronic, relapsing pattern, with many people recovering on their own without formal treatment (Slutske 2006).

Phenomenologically, behavioral addictions are characterized by a craving state or urge prior to initiating the behavior, as also occurs with individuals with substance use disorders prior to substance use (Grant et al. 2013). Additionally, these behaviors are accompanied by a positive mood state or "high" in a manner similar to substance intoxication (Grant et al. 2010). Stress and emotional dysregulation may contribute to cravings in both behavioral and substance use disorders (de Castro et al. 2007). Many individuals who exhibit compulsive sexual behavior, problem gambling, kleptomania, and excessive shopping report experiencing a decrease in these positive mood states with repeated behaviors and a need to increase the intensity of the behavior to achieve the same mood effects, in a manner similar to the development of tolerance in substance addiction (Grant et al. 2006). Many people with these behavioral addictions also report a dysphoric state while abstaining from the behaviors, analogous to withdrawal (Engs 1987). Unlike substance withdrawal, however, there have been no reports of physiologically prominent or medically serious withdrawal states associated with behavioral addictions.

As with substance use disorders, financial and marital problems are common with behavioral addictions. Individuals with behavioral addictions, like those with substance addictions, will frequently commit illegal acts, such as theft, embezzlement, and writing bad checks, to either fund their addictive behavior or cope with the consequences of the behavior (Ledgerwood et al. 2007).

Limited data exist on comorbidity of substance and behavioral addictions (Grant 2008). Several epidemiological studies support a relationship between pathological gambling and substance use disorders. The highest correlation was observed between gambling, alcohol use disorders, and antisocial personality disorder. Studies in clinical samples also suggest strong co-occurrence between substance use disorders and behavioral addictions (Grant 2008).

Another line of evidence arguing for a common substrate in both substance and behavioral addictions comes from treatment studies. First, a common treatment strategy in behavioral addictions, as in substance use disorders, is engagement in 12-step programs (Toneatto and Dragonetti 2008). Furthermore, there is accumulating evidence that these conditions respond to cognitive-behavioral therapy techniques modeled along relapse prevention strategies originally developed for substance use disorders (Aboujaoude and Koran 2010; Mitchell et al. 2006; Petry et al. 2006). There is currently no medication approved for any of the behavioral addictions. However, opioid antagonists, such as naltrexone, have been found to reduce drive to engage in addictive behaviors such as pathological gambling and kleptomania (Grant and Kim 2002; Kim 1998). Engs (1987) presented a list of the common characteristics of addictive behaviors (Table 2–1).

These similarities between behavioral addictions and substance use addictions are presented primarily to discuss the concerns of Brent Colasurdo in his legal treatise "Behavioral Addictions and the Law" (Colasurdo 2010) in which he concluded that

> Using the addiction label for patterns of excessive, self-destructive behavior has the potential to create confusion and anomalous results in the legal system. Currently, there is little empirical data supporting the ascription of mental disorder status on behavioral addictions. In contrast, chemicals create measurable withdrawal and tolerance effects that gave rise to the concept of addiction. Although these effects do not make the concept of addiction simple or clear cut, they at least provide a quantifiable basis on which to define the disorder. Therefore, this note recommends that in the eyes of the law, the concept of addiction be restricted to chemical substance dependence. (p. 199)

From a legal perspective, *Black's Law Dictionary* defines *intent* as "the state of mind accompanying an act, especially a forbidden act" knowing that "while motive is the inducement to do some act, intent is the mental resolution or determination to do it" and concluding that "when the intent to do an act that violates the law exists, motive becomes immaterial" (Garner 2009, p. 881). Possessing and manifesting the requisite intent for criminal or civil liability is considered to rest upon a defendant's exercise of "free will."

Barrett and Limoges (2011) observed with respect to behavioral addictions that "anything that impairs the brain must also impair the mind, and will is almost unquestionably a function of the mind" (p. 255). Despite this, courts have historically been disinclined or outright unwilling "to address the ethical and philosophical implications of biological research findings," adhering to a "general presumption" that "behavior is a consequence of free will" (Denno 1988, p. 615). Nadelhoffer and Nahmias (2011), however, declared on the basis of more recent findings that "as neuroscientists continue to demystify the mind by uncovering the neural mechanisms that undergird human thought and behavior, we will see a fundamental shift in the way people think about agency and responsibility," specifically affecting "the attitudes and judgments of legal decision makers" (p. 157).

TABLE 2–1. Common characteristics of addictive behaviors

1. Obsessing over the object, activity, or substance

2. Seeking out and engaging in the behavior even though it is causing harm

3. Compulsively engaging in the activity, performing the activity over and over even if he/she does not want to and finds it difficult to stop

4. Withdrawal symptoms upon cessation of the activity, including irritability, craving, restlessness, and depression

5. Loss of control. The person does not appear to have control as to when, how long, or how much he or she will continue the behavior

6. Person often denies problems resulting from his/her engagement in the behavior, even though others can see the negative effects

7. Person hides the behavior after family or close friends mention their concern

8. Depression and low self-esteem

Source. Extracted from Engs, Ruth C. "The pharmacology of drugs," in Alcohol and Other Drugs: Self Responsibility. Bloomington, IN, Tichenor Publishing, 1987, pp 52–53. Used by permission of the author. Available at: http://www.indiana.edu/~engs/rbook

When the legal decision making in question involves sentencing, "many believe that the modern scientific understanding of individual choice debunks the widely held assumption that human behavior is caused by an internal faculty in agents called 'free will'" (Atiq 2013, p. 449), a concept "central to retributive theories of punishment" (Chiesa 2011, p. 1403). In no arena is this played out more dramatically than in that of capital sentencing, in which "the introduction of evidence of impairment alone is not likely to be as effective when used without evidence of unsuccessful attempts to overcome the impairment" (Dickson 2009, p. 1124). Wright (2012), O'Hanlon (2009), and Littman (1997) are among the legal commentators who have grappled in the past with attempts to define the boundaries of social scientific contributions to sentencing and damages.

Colasurdo (2010) observed that "popular culture, the psychiatric community, and the legal system, have become increasingly accepting of behavioral addictions as mental disorders" (p. 163). This circumstance led Karim and Chaudhri (2012) to pose the following question:

> The concept of self-medicating with substances is well known, but how about self-medicating with behaviors? The use of repetitive actions, initiated by an impulse that can't be stopped, causing an individual to escape, numb, soothe, release tension, lessen anxiety or feel euphoric, may redefine the term addiction to include experience and not just substance. (p. 5)

There can be little argument by now, with the generally settled legal and scientific acceptance, that the answer to Holden's (2001) question, "'Behavioral' Addictions: Do They Exist?" in the high-profile journal *Science* is *yes*. The di-

lemma of the modern criminal or civil court lies in determining how far to extend these notions, transcending "conceptual presuppositions of their own
making" (Westen 2005, p. 599) in order to appreciate that while "responsibility
for conduct requires that human persons have free choice about what they do,"
legal advocates are increasingly in a position to argue that "according to physical, behavioral, or psychological deterministic accounts of human behavior—
such a demand is an impossibility" (Lyons 2007, p. 102).

DSM-5 "Cautionary Statement for Forensic Use of DSM-5"

DSM-IV-TR (American Psychiatric Association 2000) included a 19-line, approximately half-page "cautionary statement" that only in its final two sen-
tences undertook to address legal applications, asserting as follows:

> It is to be understood that inclusion here, for clinical and research purposes, of a
> diagnostic category such as Pathological Gambling or Pedophilia does not imply
> that the condition meets legal or other non-medical criteria for what constitutes
> a mental disease, mental disorder, or mental disability. The clinical and scientific
> considerations involved in categorization of these conditions as mental disor-
> ders may not be wholly relevant to legal judgments, for example, that take into
> account such issues as individual responsibility, disability determination, and
> competency. (p. xxxvii)

DSM-5 has taken a palpably more aggressive approach to the subject, with a
nonexclusive focus on legally relevant applications. The new 42-line full-page
treatment is entitled "Cautionary Statement for Forensic Use of DSM-5." It continues to refer to such behavioral addictions as "gambling disorder" and "pedo-
philic disorder" but differs from its DSM-IV-TR predecessor by virtue of the
great lengths to which it goes to disabuse criminal and civil attorneys of any notion of a direct connection between DSM-5 nosology and codified legal standards. Here one reads of "the imperfect fit between the questions of ultimate
concern to the law and the information contained in a clinical diagnosis," "the
risks and limitations" of using the DSM-5 "in forensic settings," and the importance of understanding that "the clinical diagnosis" of a disorder "does not im-
ply that an individual with such a condition meets legal criteria for the presence
of a mental disorder or a specific legal standard (e.g., for competence, criminal
responsibility, or disability)" (p. 25). With particular relevance to the legal ramifications of behavioral addictions, the following conclusion is offered:

> Nonclinical decision makers should also be cautioned that a diagnosis does not
> carry any necessary implications regarding the etiology or causes of the individ-
> ual's mental disorder or the individual's degree of control over behaviors that

may be associated with the disorder. Even when diminished control over one's behavior is a feature of the disorder, having the diagnosis in itself does not demonstrate that a particular individual is (or was) unable to control his or her behavior at a particular time. (p. 25)

Although no *necessary* causal implications are drawn from the presence of a psychiatric diagnosis and although the presence of a psychiatric diagnosis *in itself* is insufficient for establishing a defendant's possession or lack of *free will* during a specific legally relevant incident, the inclusion of this cautionary statement will do little to prevent the legal system's deliberate reliance on the contents of DSM-5.

Criminal and civil attorneys will continue to pore over these diagnostic criteria in order to obtain all of the adversarial leverage that can be gained from the fact that a doctor ascribed—or declined to ascribe—a particular label to a defendant on the basis of a codified set of functional and historical criteria. Indeed, to fail to take such foundational, commonly invoked medical standards into account would be tantamount to legal malpractice. Following are some examples of current DSM-5 diagnostic schemes, replete with analyses from a practical legal perspective.

Pyromania

A DSM-5 (p. 476) diagnosis of pyromania requires that the criminal or civil defendant meets the criteria outlined in Box 2–1.

Box 2–1. DSM-5 Criteria for Pyromania

A. Deliberate and purposeful fire setting on more than one occasion.
B. Tension or affective arousal before the act.
C. Fascination with, interest in, curiosity about, or attraction to fire and its situational contexts (e.g., paraphernalia, uses, consequences).
D. Pleasure, gratification, or relief when setting fires or when witnessing or participating in their aftermath.
E. The fire setting is not done for monetary gain, as an expression of sociopolitical ideology, to conceal criminal activity, to express anger or vengeance, to improve one's living circumstances, in response to a delusion or hallucination, or as a result of impaired judgment (e.g., in major neurocognitive disorder, intellectual disability [intellectual developmental disorder], substance intoxication).
F. The fire setting is not better explained by conduct disorder, a manic episode, or antisocial personality disorder.

Source. Reprinted from the *Diagnostic and Statistical Manual of Mental Disorders,* 5th Edition. Arlington, VA, American Psychiatric Association, 2013. Used with permission. Copyright © 2013 American Psychiatric Association.

Despite the mania component of this label, one can see that these criteria bespeak anything but a frenzied loss of control, and, indeed, the presence of a manic episode as the most compelling basis for this type of fire-setting behavior is specified as a reason that the defendant would not qualify for a diagnosis of pyromania. The same is clearly being said of those who lack *free will* because of what until recently would have been described as mental retardation or because of command hallucinations or other manifestations of psychosis.

It is not only capacity-driven notions of involuntariness that would call for a differential diagnosis when pyromania is being considered. Several willful mind-sets are also disqualifying, such as those that are financially, economically, politically, or criminally motivated. The inclusion of "anger" and "vengeance" might lead one to believe that a loss of free will would be implicated in disqualification, but such prospects are dimmed by the specification that acting "to express" such feelings would rule out pyromania.

Most prominent among diagnostic criteria related to free will issues is the necessary characterization of the fire-setting behavior in question as "deliberate and purposeful" for qualification as a manifestation of pyromania. This wording does not overtly suggest an incapacity for the exercise of judgment, and such qualifiers as fascination, interest, curiosity, attraction, pleasure, gratification, and relief are clearly not intended to convey any expressed notions of behavioral compulsion. DSM-5 text accompanying these criteria further refers to such dependence as potentially being "indifferent to the consequences" (p. 476) or positioned to "derive satisfaction" (p. 477), with a loss of control never being implied. Indeed, specific reference is made to the possibility that defendants who wind up qualifying for a diagnosis of pyromania "may make considerable advance preparation for starting a fire" (p. 476).

Black's Law Dictionary (Garner 2009) defines *arson* at common law as "the malicious burning of someone else's dwelling house"; modern statutory schemes tend to focus on "the intentional and wrongful burning of someone else's property (as to destroy a building) or one's own property (as to fraudulently collect insurance)" (p. 126). By way of example, Massachusetts requires a person convicted of arson to have acted "willfully and maliciously" in this regard (Mass. Gen. Laws ch. 266, §1 2013). Applying DSM-5 criteria for pyromania to this scheme, Massachusetts prosecutors would presumably have little cause to fear that this diagnosis would somehow be asserted in constituting a mental health defense to arson. Indeed, they would likely point in particular to the phrase "deliberate and purposeful" in asserting that pyromania, whatever its ultimately mitigating effect on sentencing, comports with precisely those behaviors and concurrent mental states that the statute in question is intended to address. Similarly, from a civil perspective, plaintiffs' attorneys would be in a position to argue that pyromania in no way obviates the responsibility of an individual being sued for damages that have resulted from fire setting.

Kleptomania

A DSM-5 (p. 478) diagnosis of kleptomania requires that the criminal or civil defendant meets the criteria outlined in Box 2–2.

Box 2–2.   DSM-5 Criteria for Kleptomania

A. Recurrent failure to resist impulses to steal objects that are not needed for personal use or for their monetary value.
B. Increasing sense of tension immediately before committing the theft.
C. Pleasure, gratification, or relief at the time of committing the theft.
D. The stealing is not committed to express anger or vengeance and is not in response to a delusion or a hallucination.
E. The stealing is not better explained by conduct disorder, a manic episode, or antisocial personality disorder.

Source.   Reprinted from the *Diagnostic and Statistical Manual of Mental Disorders,* 5th Edition. Arlington, VA, American Psychiatric Association, 2013. Used with permission. Copyright © 2013 American Psychiatric Association.

Similar to pyromania, kleptomania is ruled out if the defendant is found to have been responding to command hallucinations or other manifestations of psychosis, and manic episodes cannot be the source of the mania this label reflects. Behavior undertaken to express an angered or vengeful mind-set is once again a basis for diagnostic exclusion, and pleasure, gratification, and relief are not descriptors designed to inflame the imaginations of defense attorneys seeking to exculpate criminal or otherwise actionable behavior.

Notably distinct from pyromania, however, kleptomania is not described in terms of "deliberate and purposeful actions" but rather is described with respect to a "failure to resist impulses" with a sense of tension that is not just present but is, in fact, increasing. Can counsel assert that this accommodates not just a disinclination to refrain from engaging in theft but a situation in which the defendant strove to overcome such impulses in vain? The accompanying DSM-5 text is favorable to this perspective, helpfully explaining that afflicted persons "typically attempt to resist the impulse to steal, and they are aware that the act is wrong and senseless," reflecting the criterion in Box 2–2 that stolen objects "are not needed for personal use or for their monetary value" (p. 478).

Suggesting still further that such activities may reflect an erosion or even inaccessibility of control, DSM-5 further indicates that "neurotransmitter pathways associated with behavioral addictions, including those associated with the serotonin, dopamine, and opioid systems, appear to play a role in kleptomania as well" (p. 478). Here kleptomania appears to be designated as an addiction per se, and an event is regarded as on a similar biochemically driven basis as substance dependence. Furthermore, a critical distinction is made by way of the clarification that kleptomania "should be distinguished from ordinary acts of theft or shoplifting," as "ordinary theft (whether planned or impulsive) is deliberate" (p. 479). Clearly, kleptomania is being characterized as not deliberate, in stark contrast with pyromania, in which the deliberate nature of a defendant's illegal activity is the primary diagnostic criterion (p. 476).

Black's Law Dictionary (Garner 2009) defines *shoplifting* at common law as "theft of merchandise from a store of business; specifically, larceny of goods from a store or other commercial establishment by willfully taking and concealing the merchandise with the intention of converting the goods to one's personal use without paying the purchase price" (p. 1504). By way of example, Virginia requires a person convicted of shoplifting to be someone who "willfully conceals or takes possession of the goods or merchandise of any store or other mercantile establishment" (Va. Code Ann. § 18.2-103 2013). Applying DSM-5 criteria for kleptomania to this scheme, Virginia prosecutors would be faced with the potentially daunting task of establishing that a defendant legitimately diagnosed with a disorder that is not deliberate in nature could be found beyond a reasonable doubt to have been acting willfully. Similarly, from a civil perspective, plaintiffs' attorneys might find it difficult to establish that a person diagnosed with kleptomania intentionally sought to deprive another individual of goods or personal possessions.

Gambling Disorder

A DSM-5 (p. 585) diagnosis of gambling disorder—formerly, pathological gambling, as addressed in DSM-IV-TR (pp. 671–674)—requires that the criminal or civil defendant meet the criteria shown in Box 2–3.

Box 2–3.   DSM-5 Criteria for Gambling Disorder

A. Persistent and recurrent problematic gambling behavior leading to clinically significant impairment or distress, as indicated by the individual exhibiting four (or more) of the following in a 12-month period:
   1. Needs to gamble with increasing amounts of money in order to achieve the desired excitement.
   2. Is restless or irritable when attempting to cut down or stop gambling.
   3. Has made repeated unsuccessful efforts to control, cut back, or stop gambling.
   4. Is often preoccupied with gambling (e.g., having persistent thoughts of reliving past gambling experiences, handicapping or planning the next venture, thinking of ways to get money with which to gamble).
   5. Often gambles when feeling distressed (e.g., helpless, guilty, anxious, depressed).

6. After losing money gambling, often returns another day to get even ("chasing" one's losses).
7. Lies to conceal the extent of involvement with gambling.
8. Has jeopardized or lost a significant relationship, job, or educational or career opportunity because of gambling.
9. Relies on others to provide money to relieve desperate financial situations caused by gambling.

B. The gambling behavior is not better explained by a manic episode.

Specify if:
Episodic: Meeting diagnostic criteria at more than one time point, with symptoms subsiding between periods of gambling disorder for at least several months.
Persistent: Experiencing continuous symptoms, to meet diagnostic criteria for multiple years.

Specify if:
In early remission: After full criteria for gambling disorder were previously met, none of the criteria for gambling disorder have been met for at least 3 months but for less than 12 months.
In sustained remission: After full criteria for gambling disorder were previously met, none of the criteria for gambling disorder have been met during a period of 12 months or longer.

Specify current severity:
Mild: 4–5 criteria met.
Moderate: 6–7 criteria met.
Severe: 8–9 criteria met.

Source. Reprinted from the *Diagnostic and Statistical Manual of Mental Disorders,* 5th Edition. Arlington, VA, American Psychiatric Association, 2013. Used with permission. Copyright © 2013 American Psychiatric Association.

Here the component most relevant to any notion of free will would be the requirement that a defendant diagnosed with gambling disorder "has made repeated unsuccessful attempts to control, cut back, or stop gambling." This indicates that persons have tried on more than one occasion to control the problem, failing to do so not because they did not want to change but rather because they could not change without the assistance of others. Emotional states of being restless or irritable will appear considerably less compelling from a defense perspective in either criminal or civil contexts, although the reference to "desperate financial situations" may be seen as more exculpatory in nature. DSM-5 text also refers to "distortions in thinking" that are observed in conjunction with gambling disorder and observes that "up to half of individuals in treatment for gambling disorder have suicidal ideation, and about 17% have attempted suicide" (p. 587).

Gambling disorder is placed under the general DSM-5 heading "Substance-Related and Addictive Disorders" (pp. 481–589) and is the sole diagnosis to be found under the subheading "Non-Substance-Related Disorders" (pp. 585–589). Barrett and Limoges (2011) similarly labeled this disorder as one of the "addictions without substance," lamenting the fact that such maladies are "given little, if any, emphasis in professional training programs that address substance dependence" (p. 257), and they further observe that

> Learning theory is among the most relevant areas of expertise…at the present time, clinical lore and the scientific findings on the addictions without substance are in relative infancy when compared with those of alcohol and other substance abuse. Practitioners who conduct forensic assessment of addictions will do well to keep a weather eye out for this evidence. (p. 265)

Black's Law Dictionary (Garner 2009) defines *embezzlement* at common law as "the fraudulent taking of personal property with which one has been entrusted, especially as a fiduciary," noting further that "the criminal intent for embezzlement—unlike larceny and false pretenses—arises after taking possession (not before or during the taking)" (p. 599).

By way of example, Michigan requires a person convicted of embezzlement to be someone who

> fraudulently disposes of or converts to his or her own use, or takes or secretes with the intent to convert to his or her own use without the consent of his or her principal, any money or other personal property of his or her principal that has come to that person's possession or that is under his or her charge or control by virtue of his or her being an agent, servant, employee, trustee, bailee or custodian. (Mich. Comp. Laws § 750.174 2013)

In this context, the "intent" in question is again one that arises after taking possession, and the law addresses its "use" without reference to any specific reason for doing so. This would make the assertion of an outright insanity defense particularly difficult, although there would be ample opportunities for mitigation with respect to this statutory definition. In civil contexts, the fact that a defendant has made "repeated unsuccessful attempts to control" his or her gambling disorder would likely be raised during any attempt to assess appropriate damages.

Behavioral Addictions and Forensic Relationships

Here we have attempted in three areas—pyromania, kleptomania, and gambling disorder—to relate these behavioral addictions to legal concepts. Pyromania is clearly related to fire setting, and kleptomania is related to stealing or theft, but gambling disorder and embezzlement are not as clearly related. One does not necessarily embezzle when one has a gambling disorder. However, pyromania, kleptomania, and gambling disorder are related by virtue of the type of diagnosis and legal concept.

Perhaps the most common behavioral addiction that has most customarily led to criminal sanctions is gambling addiction. Persons involved in gambling may become involved in criminal behavior if they cheat at the gaming table (embezzlement?) or if they steal in order to support their habits or addictions. However, there are those involved in civil cases who claim that they should be reimbursed for their losses because of their gambling addiction, or what has been referred to in DSM-IV-TR as "pathological gambling" and is now referred to in DSM-5 as gambling disorder.

One particular case involved a man who lost over $2 million at the casinos in Las Vegas. He sued to have the money restored to him because he alleged that the owners of the casino "knew, or should have known" that he had a gambling addiction and should not have loaned him money or allowed him to borrow and then lose even more. He claimed that his condition was one that is uncontrollable for him, and the owners of the casino took advantage of his mental infirmity. On examination, he was asked whether he ever had a "big win," which many gambling addicts do have and which encourages them to continue. He responded that he had won half a million dollars in one particular evening several years before. When asked whether he gave the money back, he said, "Of course not, why should I?" The examiner responded "for the same reason you are asking the owners to reimburse you for their 'big win' from you." He understood the relationship and recognized that he would have no legal ground to stand on because he was asking the casino to do something that he would not have done himself, and he was clearly aware that he had a gambling problem. Other gambling addicts have fared worse by not being able to pay their debt and having to declare bankruptcy or being threatened by loan sharks who they approached in order to continue their addictive behavior.

Another major area in forensic work with behavioral addictions is that relating to pyromania. One often sees the fire setter as one who had early experiences of fascination with fire. This fascination goes beyond the accidental burning of a field or the child's curiosity about flames. The repetitive behavior of setting small fires and being fascinated (and often sexually excited) by the fire is the determining factor. Some of these individuals choose to become firefighters in order to put out the fires that fascinate them. We have seen a number of cases in which the fire setters were firefighters who rationalized that their departments were not busy enough and needed not only experience in putting out fires but also public attention in order to affirm their real value to the community by saving lives and property. Mostly, the fires they set involved empty buildings in which no one was hurt. However, there are those who set fires without regard to the lives of others who may be trapped in the building and who may perish in the flames. Clearly, these are criminal legal matters that need to be resolved through the criminal justice system. However, these individuals may also become involved in civil litigation for restitution of the property they destroyed.

Another major forensic relationship to behavioral addiction is that of kleptomania, or stealing for no particular purpose. Related to kleptomania is the behavioral addiction of excessive buying. There are those who can afford to buy and who store what they buy without ever opening the package. People who have behavioral addictions related to taking or buying will often take merchandise without paying for it. This is known as kleptomania. Others will pay for what they buy and receive satisfaction from collecting more material goods than they could ever use. People with manic depressive disorder, when in a manic phase, often buy excessively and run into financial difficulties, being unable to afford what they have bought. Others will steal excessively in a manic phase. It is clear that many of these behavioral addictions do not exist by themselves but are related to major mental disorders such as bipolar disorder, major depressive disorder, or schizophrenia.

When it comes to hoarding, another behavioral addiction, police have often found large caches of worthless paper and spoiled foodstuffs when searching the homes of criminal defendants. In one such case, the odor was particularly horrendous; when the police entered the home, they found spoiled cheese, eggs, and milk that were never consumed, were collected over the years, and were never refrigerated. Other hoarders include those who collect animals; they are unable to care for these animals, but they will collect as many as they can. They may be charged with cruelty to animals. One woman with kleptomania was later arrested, and the police found stored in her home 400 boxes of shoes that she had taken from various stores, several hundred dresses, scores of underwear, and dozens of socks. She had never opened most of the packages, and did not wear the garments, but stole for the thrill of taking, not of using.

One of the more recently identified behavioral disorders is Internet addiction. There are those who are addicted to the Internet and spend hours and hours at a time sitting in front of the computer, collecting data and information and searching new avenues for information. There are others who use the Internet for stalking or intimidating or "cyber bullying." Some will become legally involved for crossing the boundary between personal use and disturbing the peace of others.

One of the most common legal problems noted with Internet addiction is the pedophile who repeatedly downloads child pornography. There have been several cases of individuals who have downloaded child pornography through international Internet activity and who have distributed and traded pictures of children involved in sexual activity. Many of these men do not act on their interest in sex with children but confine themselves to the vicarious pleasure of looking at pictures and videos. However, the production of such videos is harmful to children, and those who engage in this business are considered criminal for encouraging the abuse of children.

There are also those who utilize the Internet in order to meet young girls for sexual purposes. A number of men have corresponded by Internet with females who claim to be 12, 13, or 14 years of age but, in fact, are federal, state, and local law enforcement agents seeking to arrest those who would meet with and have sex with minors.

This latter group falls under the category of sexual addiction, which is also clearly a behavioral addiction with forensic implications. There are a number of men and women who claim to be "hypersexual," primarily when they are in a hypomanic or manic phase of bipolar disorder. Some do not have a bipolar diagnosis; they are predators who seek out women in bars and other places, giving them date rape drugs in order to intoxicate them and render them unconscious to take advantage of them sexually. For most of these men, their addiction is confined to sexual behavior, but some go beyond that and kill their victims after sexually abusing them. Some men have an antipathy toward prostitutes and will seek prostitutes on the street in order to punish them for their criminal and lewd behavior. At the far extreme of sexual addiction is the serial rapist-murderer.

Another area of behavioral addiction and the law involves *workaholics*— people who have an addiction to work and feel compelled to work as much as they are able. Examination of individuals of this type who become involved in legal matters find that the addiction is often related to bipolar disorder and that the individual in a manic phase may brag about working 72 hours in a row without sleep and without rest, a violation of laws that regulate work hours.

There are workplace behaviors that become forensic issues, especially when discrimination and harassment occur in the workplace. Employees have complained that their supervisors at work harass them sexually and occasionally demand sex even in the office or after work in order for the employee to maintain his or her employment. If the sexual advances occur without consent or under duress, the supervisor may be charged in criminal court with rape or sexual assault. Even with those behavioral addictions not normally associated with forensic issues, there may be legal consequences to the behaviors. For example, excessive exercising may result in the loss of employment because the individual is late for work or misses work because of the excessive time taken to exercise. The person may plead that he or she could not attend to their work because of the obsession with exercise.

With respect to food addiction, there may be civil forensic issues for a person who is so anorexic or bulimic that he or she loses weight and cannot go to work because of his or her illness, because of vomiting, because of lack of energy, or because of a very thin appearance and his or her wish not to be seen by others.

On the other hand, the individual may be so addicted to food that he or she gains an enormous amount of weight and cannot function at work. The issue would then be the grounds for a disability finding or an administrative hearing because of a behavioral addiction that led to a mental or physical disability.

Similarly, with respect to tanning, the individual may be so addicted to tanning that he or she develops skin cancer or other ailments that may lead to a disability, an inability to work, or even a lawsuit for negligence on the part of the tanning organization.

Also, those addicted to the Internet may misuse their privileges at work by abusing the computers at work, using the computers for personal rather than work efforts. They may also be so addicted to the Internet that they miss or are late for work.

There are those who have criticized the use of behavioral addictions in legal proceedings. Colasurdo (2010) pointed out that currently there are few empirical data supporting the description of mental disorder status of behavioral addictions. In contrast, chemicals create measurable withdrawal effects that can substantiate the concept of addiction. Colasurdo concluded that the concept of addiction should be restricted to chemical substance dependence.

Conclusion

We have seen that there are a number of forensic implications to behavioral addictions that may involve fairly innocent behaviors such as tanning, exercise, and eating, but it is more likely that traditional behavioral addictions, such as kleptomania, pyromania, gambling addiction, Internet addiction, and sexual addiction, will result in forensic consequences of a civil or criminal nature. The law demands that free will be considered as an issue in gauging criminal behavior: Was the person acting deliberately or willfully? Some of the behavioral addictions preclude total voluntary, deliberate, purposeful, and willing behavior. It is those addictions that can be discussed by the forensic mental health expert in terms of competency, disability, and criminal responsibility. Clearly, such conditions will be relevant to sentencing in criminal behaviors when the degree of responsibility is diminished by the behavioral addiction.

Questions for the future involve the neuroscientific, genetic, and other chemical or neurochemical bases for the behavioral addictions. These may have similar import to the bases for substance use disorders.

References

Aboujaoude E, Koran LM: Impulse Control Disorders. New York, Cambridge University Press, 2010

American Psychiatric Association: Diagnostic and Statistical Manual of Mental Disorders, 4th Edition, Text Revision. Washington, DC, American Psychiatric Association, 2000

American Psychiatric Association: Diagnostic and Statistical Manual of Mental Disorders, 5th Edition. Arlington, VA, American Psychiatric Association, 2013

Atiq EH: How folk beliefs about free will influence sentencing: a new target for the neuro-determinist critics of criminal law. New Criminal Law Review 16:449–493, 2013

Barrett CL, Limoges RF: Addictions, in Handbook of Forensic Assessment: Psychological and Psychiatric Perspectives. Edited by Drogin EY, Dattilio FM, Sadoff RL, Gutheil TG. Hoboken, NJ, Wiley, 2011, pp 255–274

Black DW: Behavioural addictions as a way to classify behaviours. Can J Psychiatry 58(5):249–251, 2013 23756284

Chambers RA, Potenza MN: Neurodevelopment, impulsivity, and adolescent gambling. J Gambl Stud 19(1):53–84, 2003 12635540

Chiesa LE: Punishing without free will. Utah Law Rev 2011:1403–1460, 2011

Colasurdo BS: Behavioral addictions and the law. South Calif Law Rev 84:161–199, 2010

de Castro V, Fong T, Rosenthal RJ, et al: A comparison of craving and emotional states between pathological gamblers and alcoholics. Addict Behav 32(8):1555–1564, 2007 17174480

Denno DW: Human biology and criminal responsibility: free will or free ride? Univ Pa Law Rev 137:615–671, 1988

Dickson M: Dismantling the free will fairytale: the importance of demonstrating the inability to overcome in death penalty narratives. UMKC Law Rev 77:1123–1146, 2009

Engs R: Alcohol and Other Drugs: Self Responsibility. Bloomington, IN, Tichenor Publishing,1987

Frascella J, Potenza MN, Brown LL, et al: Shared brain vulnerabilities open the way for nonsubstance addictions: carving addiction at a new joint? Ann N Y Acad Sci 1187:294–315, 2010 20201859

Garner BA (ed): Black's Law Dictionary, 9th Edition. St. Paul, MN, West, 2009

Grant JE: Impulse Control Disorders: A Clinician's Guide to Understanding and Treating Behavioral Addictions. New York, WW Norton, 2008

Grant, JE, Kim, SW: An open-label study of naltrexone in the treatment of kleptomania. J Clin Psychiatry, 63(4):349–356, 2002 12000210

Grant JE, Brewer JA, Potenza MN: The neurobiology of substance and behavioral addictions. CNS Spectr 11(12):924–930, 2006 17146406

Grant JE, Potenza MN, Weinstein A, et al: Introduction to behavioral addictions. Am J Drug Alcohol Abuse 36(5):233–241, 2010 20560821

Grant JE, Schreiber LR, Odlaug BL: Phenomenology and treatment of behavioural addictions. Can J Psychiatry 58(5):252–259, 2013 23756285

Holden C: 'Behavioral' addictions: do they exist? Science 294(5544):980–982, 2001 11691967

Karim R, Chaudhri P: Behavioral addictions: an overview. J Psychoactive Drugs 44(1):5–17, 2012 22641961

Kim SW: Opioid antagonists in the treatment of impulse-control disorders. J Clin Psychiatry 59(4):159–164, 1998 9590665

Ledgerwood DM, Weinstock J, Morasco BJ, et al: Clinical features and treatment prognosis of pathological gamblers with and without recent gambling-related illegal behavior. J Am Acad Psychiatry Law 35(3):294–301, 2007 17872548

Littman RJ: Adequate provocation, individual responsibility, and the deconstruction of free will. Albany Law Rev 60:1127–1170, 1997

Lyons EC: All the freedom you can want: the purported collapse of the problem of free will. J Civil Rights Economic Dev 22(1):100–164, 2007

Mass. Gen. Laws ch. 266, §1 (2013)

Mich. Comp. Laws § 750.174 (2013)

Mitchell JE, Burgard M, Faber R, et al: Cognitive behavioral therapy for compulsive buying disorder. Behav Res Ther 44(12):1859–1865, 2006 16460670

Nadelhoffer T, Nahmias E: Neuroscience, free will, folk institutions, and the criminal law. Thurgood Marshall Law Rev 36:157–176, 2011

O'Hanlon S: Towards a more reasonable approach to free will in criminal law. Cardozo Public Law, Policy and Ethics Journal 7:395–427, 2009

Petry NM, Ammerman Y, Bohl J, et al: Cognitive-behavioral therapy for pathological gamblers. J Consult Clin Psychol 74(3):555–567, 2006 16822112

Slutske WS: Natural recovery and treatment-seeking in pathological gambling: results of two U.S. national surveys. Am J Psychiatry 163(2):297–302, 2006 16449485

Toneatto T, Dragonetti R: Effectiveness of community-based treatment for problem gambling: a quasi-experimental evaluation of cognitive-behavioral vs. twelve-step therapy. Am J Addict 17(4):298–303, 2008 18612885

Va. Code Ann. § 18.2-103 (2013)

Westen P: Getting the fly out of the bottle: the false problem of free will and determinism. Buffalo Criminal Law Review 8:599–652, 2005

Wright RG: Criminal law and sentencing: what goes with free will? Drexel Law Review 5:1–48, 2012

PART II

The Behavioral Addictions

CHAPTER 3

Problematic Exercise

A Case of Alien Feet

Elias Dakwar, M.D.

IN this chapter, we examine exercise-related behaviors that resemble addiction. Like most of the other "addictions" that are discussed later in the book, however, the diagnosis of "exercise addiction" does not actually exist—that is, it is not listed in DSM-5 (American Psychiatric Association 2013) or other diagnostic references. It is also unclear if addictive processes are implicated in even a fraction of cases of problematic exercise. So why have a chapter, or an entire book for that matter, devoted to phenomena that at best are unrecognized as disorders and at worst do not even exist?

It will become clearer over the course of this chapter that exercise addiction might, indeed, be the most appropriate way to classify certain behaviors, however rare they might be. Clinicians should therefore be prepared to consider and address exercise addiction, even if those in the field have yet to understand such crucial preliminaries as how a proper diagnosis might be made. Cases like that of Jason, in which exercise is pursued in a problematic way, can be illustrative in this regard. This case can also clarify the diagnostic process whereby the differential diagnosis is systematically reduced to the most compelling explanation.

Before we delve into the case of Jason, we examine some key concepts, including addiction, reward, and exercise. This may help us better evaluate whether or not exercise addiction is the most appropriate label to apply to Jason's problematic behavior.

Addiction, Reward, and Exercise

Addiction can be most broadly defined as reward-seeking behavior that is pursued despite the emergence of various problems and that is characterized by progressive loss of self-control. The reward in the case of substance use disorders (SUDs) is engendered by drugs, such as alcohol, tobacco, or opioids. A drug-addicted individual will compulsively seek out the drug-related reward even at the cost of health and proper functioning. Behavioral addictions, on the other hand, are thought to involve nondrug rewards, such as a win in gambling, and may similarly lead to seemingly uncontrollable reward seeking, with mounting psychosocial and medical problems (Ries et al. 2009).

Reward can be operationally defined as a stimulus (such as food, sex, drugs) with hedonic salience. What exactly constitutes a reward and how a reward correlates with neurobiological processes are questions that continue to be investigated. The popular conception of reward as mediated by a direct causal relationship between a stimulus (e.g., cocaine) and dopaminergic activity in the nucleus accumbens and ventral tegmental area is now recognized as inadequate, with growing evidence suggesting a role for conditioning, neural plasticity, prefrontal regulation, other neurotransmitters, and contextual factors in reward sensitivity. Thus, the notion of a reward center that, once activated, produces a dopaminergic quantum of pleasure is obsolete (Galanter and Kleber 2008; Volkow et al. 2011).

Certain neurobiological processes, nonetheless, seem to be consistently involved in a variety of reward-related stimuli, such as drugs and natural rewards. These processes include dopaminergic, opioid, glutamatergic, and endocannabinoid circuits. This overlap between natural reward processes and those involving drug-related rewards is important to emphasize because it represents an important framework by which to understand how the problematic pursuit of natural rewards may come to resemble SUDs.

Exercise, particularly when vigorous, has also been found to produce substantial activations in reward-related circuits (Boecker et al. 2008; Dietrich and McDaniel 2004). According to the American Committee on Sports Medicine, *exercise* is physical activity, pursued at work or during leisure time, that involves mild to robust elevations in heart rate and breathing (American College of Sports Medicine 2009). There are universal recommendations for the minimum amount of moderate or vigorous exercise, by time and frequency, that should be undertaken to optimize physical (and possibly mental) health, but no guidelines currently exist on what constitutes excessive or problematic exercise. This may be a question best answered on an individual basis, as with any assessment of whether or not a behavior has begun to interfere with other aspects of life.

How can exercise be possibly problematic? Unlike drugs, gambling, or even sex, the pursuit of exercise is not generally met with criticism, moral judgment, or negative social consequences. Far from being illegal or suggestive of a poor character, exercise is highly valued. Athletes are celebrated; physical fitness is esteemed. Furthermore, the dangers and risks of exercise are negligible compared with those of drugs. In fact, not only can exercise feel good, but it is clearly good for you: reports emerge weekly indicating that regular exercise may be beneficial for depression, perhaps cancer, and a host of other medical problems. Exercise is accorded an important place in our society as a healthy and admirable activity, and it seems dissonant and absurd to classify a daily jogger with a regular cocaine user.

These factors are important to consider because they contribute to the fact that the threshold for concern with exercise is higher than with more risky activities or with substances of abuse. The ways in which exercise might become problematic, and may resemble addictive disorders, will become clearer as we review and discuss the case of Jason, which is modeled on a real patient encounter.

Clinical Case

An Introduction to Jason

Jason is a 38-year-old white man who presents to an outpatient clinic in a large metropolitan hospital seeking treatment for heroin use. He has been injecting 8–10 bags of heroin daily since age 22, with a 2-year period in his early 30s when he was on methadone maintenance. During that period of agonist treatment, he continued to inject heroin but at reduced amounts. He meets criteria for an opioid use disorder. His hope is to be fully abstinent from opioids, but he is worried about the effect that complete abstention would have on the chronic pain in his lower extremities.

At the time of the interview, Jason is an unemployed painter who obtains drugs primarily by serving as a drug courier, receiving a bundle (10 bags of heroin) for every three deliveries he makes; he keeps a bundle and then sells the rest. "I'm fast, so I make at least four bundles a day. We're talking $400 a day, on top of the bundle I get for myself." He is also receiving a monthly disability check for a foot injury he sustained en route to work as a painter 10 years ago. "I'm comfortable, I have no complaints, and that's what scares me."

He is coming to treatment at the present time because he has realized "everything was perfectly in place for [him] to keep doing this until [he] died or was busted," and the thought terrifies him. He is a well-known courier who is trusted by both the dealer and the community. It is only a matter of time, he feels, before the police or other dealers will catch on. "I need to break out of this cycle before it breaks me."

Jason discloses, however, that he may have an easier time giving up heroin than he would stopping his work as a drug courier. "It's not the money, though that is, of course, part of it. I just can't imagine giving up the running. I've always been a runner, and it's great to run and at the same time make a living of it. Maybe I should look into running legal things around."

Jason estimates that he runs approximately 30 miles a day: "If I'm using my legs, I'm running. Even if I weren't working, I'd be running, running in circles, running my feet to the bone. And the great thing about this gig is that I have a destination; I have something to take and something to give, with drugs and money waiting at the finish line."

Heroin is Jason's drug of choice, but he has used or experimented with a variety of substances, including cocaine, cannabis, methamphetamine, psychedelics, and alcohol. He also smokes cigarettes, one half pack per day, and has been doing so since age 18. He believes he may have had a drinking problem in college, when he was binge drinking every few nights and getting into trouble academically and legally. He has also ended up in the hospital on a few occasions because he was found unresponsive outside of a bar or party, covered in vomit. His drinking subsided after he began to use opioids.

"It started with pills that I was given after injuring myself, some sports injury, and I was off to the races, snorting them, smoking them, whatever increased the high. It was only a matter of time before I was mainlining heroin."

Jason enjoyed opioids initially because they gave him increased energy, pain relief, and euphoria. He also found that they heightened the exhilaration he would feel after an intense run. "I'd never felt anything like it; it's like runner's high times a thousand."

Jason's current pattern of heroin use involves keeping his "works" on him and injecting a bag or two at a time several times a day, generally right before he embarks on a particularly long run to or from a delivery. "I've learned how to keep myself at that sweet spot between feeling doped up and feeling ready to take on the world. I forget about the pain in my legs, in my feet; I forget about everything except the thrill of watching the world fly by."

Important Points

Before we continue with the case, we should summarize and discuss some important points. From the information presented thus far, we can conclude that Jason carries two diagnoses: opioid use disorder, current, and alcohol use disorder, in remission. He may also have a tobacco use disorder, although this requires further exploration. Another area requiring further exploration is comorbid psychopathology, which tends to be highly prevalent in individuals with SUDs.

As for his running, there is insufficient information at present to draw any conclusions, although there are some concerning points meriting further exploration. While exercise seems to be bound up with his drug use and the lifestyle it necessitates, it also appears to be a pleasurable pursuit in its own right—so pleasurable, in fact, that he worries it may be even more difficult to stop than heroin. The amount of running that he engages in, around 30 miles a day, also seems excessive, particularly in the presence of the lower-extremity injuries and pain to which he alludes. Furthermore, Jason emphasizes the subjective pleasure derived from running rather than any health or athletic benefits it might confer. What drives him to run, it seems, is the exhilaration and "high" he achieves, the more intense the better.

In summary, what is worth noting at this point is that Jason has an extraordinary interest in running, that he engages in it quite a bit, that he suspects he may not be able to stop if needed, and that he may be incurring physical or other problems because of it. In addition, Jason has at least two SUDs, which may represent a vulnerability to other types of addictions. Although these characteristics are quite suggestive, they do not indicate that Jason is addicted to exercising. Various aspects of his running require further exploration before such a conclusion can be considered.

The first step is to better characterize the running behavior. This will cover many of the same bases that a drug history does, but with running, of course, as the focus. This includes obtaining a better history of when he first began running, how often he was doing it initially, what he enjoyed about running, and whether his engagement in running has changed over the years. Much like a drug history, it is also important to obtain information about cravings, tolerance, withdrawal, whether running has interfered with other aspects of life, problems directly attributable to running, and prior experience, if any, with giving up running. These are important to ascertain in the absence of a standardized rubric by which to diagnose "exercise addiction." The more closely the running history parallels that of an SUD, the better a case can be made that this might be an addictive process. This approach of modifying SUD criteria to make them more relevant to a particular behavior is the best way at present for diagnosing behavioral addictions. (The only exception is pathological gambling, discussed in Chapter 5, "Gambling," which is recognized by DSM-5 and has its own criteria.)

It is also critical, of course, to investigate whether other psychiatric disorders might better explain the problematic exercise (Sadock and Sadock 2009). These include externalizing disorders associated with increased activity, such as bipolar disorder and attention-deficit/hyperactivity disorder, as well as disorders that may involve increased activity as a compensatory or neutralizing behavior, such as bulimia nervosa or obsessive-compulsive disorder.

In clarifying the impact of a psychiatric disorder on problematic exercise, we pay close attention to how the exercise behavior and the psychiatric disorder overlap. Is the excessive exercise episodic and roughly coinciding with alterations in mood and energy? This suggests a bipolar disorder. Is the excessive exercise one of many manifestations of chronic hyperactivity, with exercise-related reward not privileged over other rewards? Attention-deficit/hyperactivity disorder should be considered. Is there a pattern of overeating (bingeing) alternating with excessive exercise to counter the caloric burden (purging)? This indicates that the problem is bulimia nervosa. Alternatively, as might occur in obsessive-compulsive disorder, is the exercise a compulsive activity that serves to diminish the force of certain obsessions? Patients may also be dually diagnosed, of course, with the behavioral addiction coinciding with other psychiatric disorders. For example, a patient may have bipolar disorder and also maintain a consistently high level of problematic exercise, perhaps meriting a separate diagnosis.

As we return to the case of Jason, we give particular attention to these issues, obtaining a better history of Jason's running as well as of co-occurring psychiatric disorders.

Back to the "Hamster Wheel"

Jason was asked to elaborate on his running history.

"I've always been a runner, ever since I was a kid. I told you already about the rush and the intensity. But I also like how focused it is, how you can shut everything out. Whatever was going on at home, whatever was on my mind, I could leave that all behind when I hit the road."

With his father having left home before Jason can remember and his single mother struggling to make ends meet and raise two children while also struggling with alcoholism, Jason remembered his childhood as painful and neglectful. He would leave to go running at every opportunity as a way to escape the stress at home but also as a way to cope with the difficult feelings and thoughts he was experiencing.

"Some of the guys hanging around the house were creepy. And I mean pedophile creepy. I think one of them may even have fondled me, you know, but I can't really remember that very well. I just remember being scared, walking on eggshells all the time, worried about I don't know what....Part of the problem was how out of control everyone was. Booze was everywhere. It always felt like something was about to blow up, a fight, screaming, whatever. I wanted to run away, I wanted everything to change. I hated it all. But I didn't say anything. Too scared probably. God, I couldn't stand to be at home. I got out, went running, whenever I could."

Beginning at age 10, Jason would run to and from school, as well as run through the neighborhood after school. "I'm guessing I ran about 10 miles a day, easy. And as I started running on the track team during high school, it probably went up to 15 to 20 miles a day. I kept pushing myself harder and harder, loving the way I would feel after an intense go at it. My head swimming, my limbs all warm and jelly. And there was this insane sense of power. I would feel like nothing could touch me, that I was king of the world."

Jason entered college with the intention of continuing to run track, but he was kicked off the team a few months into his freshman semester for repeatedly coming to practice drunk. "I began to drink and smoke pot in high school, but that really took off in college, particularly drinking. I would drink to black out on the weekends and would have a few beers or a few shots every other day of the week."

"Would I drink and run? Sure. It wasn't a consistent thing, but it would happen. Listen, they wanted me off the team because I wouldn't follow orders. I didn't need people to tell me how to run; I'd been doing it all my life. My coming drunk was just to piss them off. I didn't really like to run drunk, what with stumbling all over myself and feeling stupid. Booze is much better after a run, not while you're actually running. It's not like dope, which gives you the high and keeps you running all at the same time."

During his junior year, Jason tore a ligament in his knee when he took a misstep while running and landed on a hyperextended leg. "My coaches had always warned me that I would hurt myself one day. They had all sorts of comments about how I wouldn't pace myself properly, that my gait was sloppy, that I wasn't careful about my landings. That was one of my main issues with the whole sports thing. Running was my life, what I enjoyed more than anything else, not some performance that you can tweak. One guy even said it seemed that it was my goal to wear my body out as much as possible. He's right, but not in the way he thought. The more I punished my body, the higher I would fly."

"Anyway, there I was with this torn ligament, and I was told not to run and let it heal, and I was going out of my mind stir-crazy. I couldn't stop thinking about how amazing it felt to have the open road in front of you and the wind at your back. I think I even started to feel depressed, not wanting to do anything."

"I held off for maybe a few days before I was running again, gobbling up the pills to keep me going. The pills helped quite a bit; in fact, I felt even better after a run than ever before. It was like the fuel I needed. But after a week or so, no amount of pills could fix things, my knee had swollen up to the size of a grapefruit, and I could barely walk. They had to operate."

"Those few days before and after the surgery were terrible. I had never felt so messed up in my life, almost suicidal. I was in a brace, I had to walk with crutches, and I felt as if my body was shutting down. The only thing that helped was the pills, and I started using more and more of them. I loved the ecstasy and warmth and absolute peace, and I'm sure you've heard it all before. Within a few weeks of the surgery, I had started snorting and smoking them and fishing around for where I might find more."

Jason further relates that he began to run again a month or so after the surgery, well before he was advised to do so by his physicians. "I didn't care. I needed to be back on my feet. And by this point, I was using so many pills that nothing could touch me. It was funny how at first even a little running would get my head flying. Perhaps it was the pills, or maybe I was out of shape, but in that first week, a few miles would do for me what several miles had done previously."

Jason was back within a month to running close to 20 miles a day. His opioid use also continued to intensify. He stopped going to classes, and his grades suffered. "College wasn't really for me in the first place. I didn't know what I wanted to do with my life, and I found the parties boring. I didn't have many friends; I wasn't really interested in any of the girls. I was very much a loner, and I think everyone knew that. People left me alone. As long as I had my drugs and free time to do what I wanted, I was happy."

"Look, do I wish I had done more with my time back then instead of running and popping pills and whatever? Sure, why not. Perhaps I would have met a good wife, got a degree, whatever. But that's not the direction my life took."

Jason dropped out of college in his junior year, began to inject heroin shortly thereafter, and took up work as a painter. "That was also doomed from the start. I found the work boring, with too much standing around. I would have much rather been running around, you know, like I do now. But it paid the bills, and though I knew it had an expiration date, I did a half-assed job, just good enough to keep getting asked back, until the foot thing happened."

Though he was able to pass it off as a work-related injury in order to receive compensation, Jason had developed at age 28 bone spurs in his right heel, bilateral plantar fasciitis, and inflammation of the sesamoid bones in his left foot—all directly attributable to his running. These various ailments led him to stop working, but they did not prevent him from running. "Sure I may have made things worse by continuing to run. And I realize how crazy it must sound that I continued to run and continued to increase the intensity of my runs, even as my feet were falling apart. At some level, I knew I should give it a break, let my body heal. But I couldn't stop, and unless you're a devoted runner, you wouldn't understand. I needed to run like I needed to breathe.

"But I started thinking about what had happened before, with my knee blowing up like that and needing surgery, and I didn't want the same thing to happen. So I started getting into supplements and gait training and things like that to make sure that my feet were taken care of. I bought new shoes, top-of-the-line running shoes, nearly every month. I would do odd jobs, rely on the disability checks. Sometimes I didn't have enough to eat, between buying the heroin and the running supplies, but I made it happen. This drug running thing was a godsend…or a deal with the devil, depending on how you look at it. But things have been easy, maybe too easy, for the past year or so."

"And there have been good days and bad days, but my feet haven't really deteriorated much over the past few years. Then again, I haven't been off dope long enough to know the extent of the damage. I mean, I may not be feeling too much pain, but it doesn't take a foot surgeon to know that my feet don't look good, more alien than human. No toenails, the little bones all misplaced, you get the picture."

"Do I think my running is a problem? Would I rather be able to run like a normal person, a few laps around the reservoir and call it a day? Sure. But it's not easy when everything is set up to keep me running, delivering, and using. I need to get out of this hamster wheel, but I'm not sure how."

Except for acute dysphoria experienced during periods of inactivity, Jason denies a history of depressive symptoms. Although he experienced trauma and neglect in childhood, he also denies symptoms indicative of posttraumatic stress disorder.

He further denies a history of manic symptoms, panic, generalized anxiety, psychosis, active suicidality, obsessions, compulsions, binge eating, and phobias. He reports that he was energetic as a child but was a good student and generally well behaved. He denies any difficulties with concentration or attention emerging in childhood. There is no history of problems with shopping, sex, or gambling.

He also denies medical problems other than the running-related injuries in his feet and legs. He reports a robust appetite, despite his heroin use, and aims to eat at least 3,000 calories a day to ensure adequate nutrition.

Discussion

We now have sufficient information to determine whether the problematic exercise is best understood as an addiction-type process or as a manifestation of a separate psychiatric disorder. We are also in a better position to propose some possible treatments for Jason.

As mentioned in the section "Addiction, Reward, and Exercise," the most reasonable way to investigate whether or not Jason's problematic exercise merits the diagnosis of an addiction is to first modify DSM-5 SUD criteria so that they are targeted toward exercise and then to assess whether his exercise behavior meets these criteria.

Analyzed in this way, Jason's behavior meets many of these modified criteria. He spent a great deal of time either running or recovering from running. He experienced substantial difficulty in reducing his running or not running altogether. He experienced cravings to run, as well as withdrawal-type effects (e.g., dysphoria, restlessness) when not running; he may have also experienced *tolerance*, needing to run progressively longer distances and with greater intensity to continue obtaining the intended effect. Finally, running significantly interfered with various aspects of his life, negatively affecting work, relationships, health, and schooling. Jason continued to run despite these problems.

These latter two points are perhaps most important in differentiating avid exercisers from individuals who exercise in an addictive manner. A devoted runner, for example, may meet many of the other modified criteria, including tolerance, withdrawal, cravings, difficulty stopping, and amount of time spent running. However, unless the running significantly interferes with life and is persistently pursued, it is unlikely to represent an addictive process, even if the other criteria are met.

There are other characteristics of Jason's running behavior that reinforce the impression of an addictive process. It is important to note, first, that it was predominantly the pleasurable experience of running, and not any associated advantage such as better health, that served to motivate Jason to run. This hedonic component was what led him to begin running in the first place, and his single-mindedness reward seeking only intensified as he grew older. Another noteworthy aspect of his problematic running is that it emerged during a period of great trauma and was partly a response to the deprivations he experienced during childhood. This is a genesis story common to many addicted individuals, in which the reward of choice derives an early and momentous significance by being experienced as ameliorating life's difficulties. Similarly, the problem with opioids began when Jason was deprived of the ability to run for an extended period; he found in opioids a surrogate high that he hoped would carry him through until he was back on his feet.

The opioids, however, turned out to be more than a temporary fix; he continued to use them well after he could run again and soon thereafter developed an opioid use disorder. The complex intersections between Jason's severe opioid use disorder and his apparent exercise addiction are worth untangling.

As has become clear by now, the running was a reward in itself and was not simply a means of obtaining heroin (though it also served that purpose). Thus, we should make clear straightaway that there were two separate rewards driving

Jason, even as each accentuated the other. This is an important distinction to make for the purposes of diagnosing a separate exercise addiction. Like most dually addicted individuals, Jason found a way to effectively integrate the two addictions into a single problematic pattern of behavior.

Running may not have been purely in the service of obtaining heroin, but was he using heroin in the service of running? Jason's account strongly suggests so. As already mentioned, Jason began using opioids as a way to continue running despite otherwise debilitating injuries, with the opioid use intensifying when the injuries left him bedridden and in apparent exercise withdrawal. Later, heroin intensified Jason's runner's high, along with providing its own strong high. Heroin also allowed him to run at his preferred intensity by alleviating pain, improving energy, and increasing stamina. Jason himself seemed to regard exercise-related rewards as primary and most central to his life; he believed he would have an easier time giving up heroin than quitting running, but he worried about the effect not using opioids would have on his running-related pain. Thus, he found himself trapped in a situation in which he runs to get heroin so that he can continue running, with no clear way out of the "hamster wheel."

Recent research suggests that the same vulnerabilities in reward-related neurocircuitry that predispose individuals to drug dependence may also result in intense engagement in exercise (Mathes et al. 2010). This may be due to the overlapping neurobiological effects of vigorous exercise and of substances of abuse, with vulnerable individuals more likely to find such rewards highly reinforcing and to pursue them aggressively (Dakwar et al. 2012). Although this is an area of study that is still quite preliminary, it provides a valuable framework for clarifying how behavioral addictions might emerge and how they might be treated, as well as a framework for understanding the high rates of co-occurrence between behavioral and substance addictions.

Treatment

Unfortunately, little research exists to guide the evidence-based treatment of disordered exercise. Therefore, we must rely on the examples of evidence-based treatments for related disorders—such as binge eating, problem gambling, and SUDs—for help in formulating an appropriate treatment.

Lack of insight and of motivation are common problems encountered in any addiction. The individual may not regard the behavior as a problem and may not be motivated to change. These challenges may be particularly pronounced in cases where the problem reward is culturally valued or associated with certain benefits, as with exercise, intimacy, or work. It can be difficult enough for individuals addicted to noxious substances, such as alcohol, to recognize they have a problem. How much greater is the difficulty when the addiction involves an activity that is widely praised and valued or with which the individual strongly identifies? Motivational interviewing is a critical first step in such situations. It may help the addicted individual to develop a broader perspective on the problem activity, acknowledging both the benefits and problems associated with it, as well as recognizing the need for change.

As with most other cases where a natural reward is pursued addictively, an abstinence-based approach is unlikely to be helpful for exercise addiction, if not impossible to implement. The challenge is to introduce more moderation and functionality into the reward-seeking behavior. This may involve behavioral strategies aimed at promoting healthier patterns of thought, emotion, and action, as well as pharmacological methods that are intended to diminish the reinforcing salience of the reward.

Cognitive-behavioral therapy has been found to be helpful for various disorders similar to exercise addiction, such as binge eating, problem gambling, and SUDs, and remains a standard manualized therapy for addressing addictive processes in the individual setting. The focus of this approach is to identify automatic thoughts that might lead to the problem behavior ("If I don't go for a run now, I'm going to feel terrible"), to supplant them with healthier thoughts, and to deliberately cultivate behavioral habits that disrupt problematic thoughts and the target behavior. Another psychotherapy strategy is mindfulness training. *Mindfulness* refers to the capacity for accepting, nonreactive, moment-to-moment attention. Rather than aiming to displace unhealthy thoughts or emotions, mindfulness training cultivates the practice of actively experiencing cognitive, physiological, or affective phenomena, however distressing they might be, with stillness, acceptance, inquisitiveness, and an awareness of their transience. Coupled with a behavioral intervention aimed at disrupting automatic patterns, mindfulness training might help addicted individuals develop a more deliberate and balanced approach to exercise.

An emerging group of pharmacotherapies is believed to benefit addiction by dampening reward salience and diminishing problematic reward-seeking behavior (Ries et al. 2009; Galanter and Kleber 2008). Naltrexone is thought to address alcohol dependence and binge eating by disrupting the contribution of endogenous opioids to reward sensitivity, and it may similarly work to attenuate the hedonic salience of exercise (Daniel et al. 1992)Daniel et al. 1992Daniel et al. 1992. Topiramate is believed to diminish the reinforcing aspects of reward by dopaminergic and γ-aminobutyric acid (GABA)–based mechanisms, and it may be helpful for alcohol and cocaine dependence, as well as binge eating. Other anticonvulsants, such as gabapentin and zonisamide, may also serve to diminish reward sensitivity. Although these medications have not been studied for problematic exercise, they exert promising antiaddiction effects and may be helpful. As with any pharmacotherapy for addiction, these medications are most likely to work in conjunction with other therapeutic supports, such as individual psychotherapy, a behavioral intervention, and groups.

Given how intertwined the two addictions are in the case of Jason, we need to address both at once in order to effectively affect either. Motivational interviewing and a behavioral intervention of some type are good places to start. As for pharmacotherapy, intramuscular naltrexone might be the most likely to provide benefit. It will likely preclude Jason from pursuing opioids, and by restoring appropriate pain sensitivity, it may encourage him to run in a more mindful manner. Similarly, a cessation of chronic analgesia may compel Jason to attend to his running-related injuries and allow his body to heal after the years of abuse. Naltrexone may also diminish the exaggerated reinforcing effects that exercise appears to have for him. Thus, naltrexone may address both the opioid and exercise addictions in one stroke. The challenge with this approach is that it necessitates detoxification, a reexperiencing of pain, and sustained abstinence from opioids. It therefore requires Jason to be fully committed to the course of treatment in anticipation of these initial hardships; this may be a hard sell given his present disinterest in experiencing pain. In accord with this approach, however, is Jason's goal of complete abstinence from opioids. Motivational interviewing oriented around this issue may be helpful at shoring up his willingness. Furthermore, delineating from the outset a course of action aimed at postdetox physical rehabilitation and pain management may promote his continued involvement with treatment.

Conclusion

This case provides an example of how problematic exercise can be approached, diagnosed, and managed. After obtaining information on Jason's running using the example of a drug history, we ascertained whether his behavior fulfilled modified SUD criteria, including an assessment of comorbid psychopathology that might better explain the behavior. Satisfied that "exercise addiction" was the most appropriate label for Jason's condition, possible treatments informed by the unique features of his case, including his co-occurring opioid dependence and pain issues, were proposed. Although exercise (and most other behavioral) addiction remains a controversial diagnosis, cases like Jason's can be helpful in beginning to understand how this type of disordered behavior might come to clinical attention, as well as how we can rely on our experience with SUDs to guide the identification and management of these related behaviors.

Key Points

- Problematic exercise can stem from a variety of psychiatric disorders, but it can also represent an addiction-type process.

- Applying modified DSM-5 criteria for substance use disorders can clarify whether or not the problematic exercise is comparable to an addiction.

- If the problematic exercise resembles addiction, it can be addressed using psychotherapy, such as cognitive-behavioral therapy, and perhaps pharmacotherapy aimed at attenuating its rewarding aspects.

References

American College of Sports Medicine: ACSM Guidelines for Exercise Testing and Prescription, 8th Edition. Philadelphia, PA, Lippincott Wiliams & Wilkins, 2009

American Psychiatric Association: Diagnostic and Statistical Manual of Mental Disorders, 5th Edition. Arlington, VA, American Psychiatric Association, 2013

Boecker H, Sprenger T, Spilker ME, et al: The runner's high: opioidergic mechanisms in the human brain. Cereb Cortex 18(11):2523–2531, 2008 18296435

Dakwar E, Blanco C, Lin KH, et al: Exercise and mental illness: results from the National Epidemiologic Survey on Alcohol and Related Conditions (NESARC). J Clin Psychiatry 73(7):960–966, 2012 22901347

Daniel M, Martin AD, Carter J: Opiate receptor blockade by naltrexone and mood state after acute physical activity. Br J Sports Med 26(2):111–115, 1992 1320440

Dietrich A, McDaniel WF: Endocannabinoids and exercise. Br J Sports Med 38(5):536–541, 2004 15388533

Galanter M, Kleber HD (eds): Textbook of Substance Abuse Treatment, 4th Edition. Washington, DC, American Psychiatric Publishing, 2008

Mathes WF, Nehrenberg DL, Gordon R, et al: Dopaminergic dysregulation in mice selectively bred for excessive exercise or obesity. Behav Brain Res 210(2):155–163, 2010 20156488

Ries R, Fiellin DA, Miller SC, et al (eds): Principles of Addiction Medicine, 4th Edition. Philadelphia, PA, Lippincott Williams & Wilkins, 2009

Sadock BJ, Sadock VA (eds): Comprehensive Textbook of Psychiatry, 9th Edition, Vol 1. Philadelphia, PA, Lippincott Williams & Wilkins, 2009

Volkow ND, Wang GJ, Fowler JS, et al: Addiction: beyond dopamine reward circuitry. Proc Natl Acad Sci USA 108(37):15037–15042, 2011 21402948

Questions

1. Which of the following medications has been shown to reduce the plea-
    sure associated with exercise?

    A. Gabapentin.
    B. Divalproex sodium.
    C. Naltrexone.
    D. Buprenorphine.
    E. Clonidine.

    The correct answer is C.

    Only naltrexone has been shown to reduce the pleasure associated with
    exercise. The mechanism is likely through antagonizing endogenous
    opioids.

2. Which one of the following is a DSM-5 disorder associated with prob-
    lematic exercise?

    A. Non-substance addiction, exercise type.
    B. Exercise addiction.
    C. Behavioral addiction, exercise type.
    D. Bulimia nervosa.
    E. Major depressive disorder.

    The correct answer is D.

    Bulimia nervosa is the only DSM-5 disorder listed that might be associ-
    ated with problematic exercise. Purging might take the form of excessive
    exercise in the disorder. Major depressive disorder is not associated with
    excessive exercise. The other disorders listed are not recognized by
    DSM-5.

3. Problematic exercise might lead to

    A. Physical debility.
    B. Withdrawal phenomena.
    C. Cravings.
    D. Occupational impairment.
    E. All of the above.

    The correct answer is E.

    All are possible complications of problematic exercise.

CHAPTER 4

Food Addiction

Sugar High

Jessica A. Gold, M.D., M.S.
Kimberly A. Teitelbaum, ARNP
Mark S. Gold, M.D.

IN our everyday speech and conversational slang, food is often labeled as "addicting." People describe having *need* for a particular food item, and even our commercial advertisements, such as the one for Pringles potato chips, suggest that "once you pop…[you can't] stop." However, despite the colloquial use of these terms, food addiction itself has been somewhat controversial in the scientific community. Yet, like other addictions with a neurobiological basis and the-oretical framework, research suggests food addiction is very much a disease and a real problem in our clinical populations.

Food addiction, like all addictions, fulfills a formal definition of disease. A patient who is addicted to food exhibits loss of control, tolerance, withdrawal, and continued use despite dangerous outcomes (Shriner and Gold 2013). This is particularly evident in the use of highly palatable foods like sugar. In a rat model, despite having access to their usual laboratory food, when provided with 2 hours of access to a sugar/fat solution, rats will consume the majority of their daily energy intake in this time period, thus exhibiting a "loss of control" (Gold 2011). These same rats will also demonstrate increased consumption after sugar abstinence and demonstrate symptoms of withdrawal, such as teeth chattering and head shakes, when given a dose of naloxone, an opioid antagonist.

Given the induced withdrawal with naloxone and other research suggesting that with overeating of palatable foods striatal dopamine D_2 receptors are downregulated and exhibit reduced sensitivity and reward (Gold 2011), it is believed that food addiction stems from the stimulation of both dopamine and μ opioid receptors (Shriner and Gold 2013). By either phasic or tonic stimulation of dopamine, sugar or other palatable foods can be both a stimulant (driving a desire to have it) and a reward (experiencing pleasure at obtaining it). Clinical disease can then exploit both the drive and reward aspects with a dual-vulnerability model. In this conceptual model, obese patients can develop a tolerance to the stimulating aspects of dopamine, but they may continue to be vulnerable to the reward aspects. Ultimately, to satisfy their drive for the reward, patients will need more and more stimulus (food) to obtain the same level of pleasure.

Yet despite similarities in clinical presentation, food addicts are not simply obese people (Shriner and Gold 2013). In fact, only 25% of participants who are obese meet the diagnostic criteria for food addiction according to the Yale Food Addiction Scale (YFAS; Avena et al. 2013), which has been shown to be clinically relevant and predictive of disease in many different populations. Using the YFAS as a guide, Table 4–1 provides a summary of the relevant screening questions a provider should ask to discern food addiction. Given that 95% of diets end in failure, clinical practitioners need to be aware that food addiction is very much a disease and, importantly, need to learn the most effective screening and treatment methods to help their patients. We hope this clinical case and the discussion that follows will help practitioners do just that.

TABLE 4–1.   Patient history: questions to ask when evaluating a person for food addiction

Does your patient

    Have control over his or her eating?

    Eat more than he or she intended?

    Drink excessive soda and sugary drinks?

    Feel addicted to fast food?

    Think about eating fatty or sugary foods multiple times a day?

    Try and fail to cut down on his or her eating?

    Gain weight despite attempts to cut down?

    Gain weight despite numerous health and life consequences?

Clinical Case

Ginger is a 62-year-old married white woman of Italian descent. She works as a hospital administrator at a local, large-volume hospital and presents to the outpatient psychiatry clinic for concerns related to her overeating and multiple diet failures. She was referred by her primary care provider, who has recommended a diet of 1,600 calories per day and has prescribed phentermine and Topamax for the patient to help suppress appetite and cravings, respectively. In the past 3 months since initiation of this regimen, Ginger has lost 2 lb in the first month and gained 4 lb in the past 2 months, for a total net gain of 2 lb. Today she expresses frustration at her lack of progress but adds, "I'm not surprised." She notes her weight has steadily risen and that in the past 40 years, she has gained 70 lb to achieve her current weight of 271 lb. Her body mass index (BMI) today is 47.

Ginger wonders if she may be addicted to food because she has tried multiple diets over her lifetime, and whereas she often loses weight initially, she has not been able to lose more than 15 lb or keep it off for more than 1 month. She states that her eating habits are poor and that while she likes fruits and vegetables and a variety of meats, she prefers carbohydrates. She also enjoys sweets and often feels a loss of control when it comes to sugary foods. Most of her eating of sugary foods is done in private. She rarely orders dessert in a restaurant but admits she will often buy cookies or cake from a grocery store and eat the entire thing on her drive home, stopping to discard the containers and receipts before arriving home. While her portions of carbohydrates are often larger than intended, her intake of sweets is "out of control." She finds it difficult to have just one cookie or one slice of cake and notes that when she starts to eat these foods, she finds herself consuming far more than intended and will even go out of her way to secure the desserts she wants from far-away bakeries or grocery stores. When her husband is away from the house, she has mixed sugar, flour, salt, and butter in a bowl and consumed the entire amount without baking it. She describes often feeling physically sick and nauseous and has eaten to the point of vomiting, but she insists that she has never intentionally purged after a binge episode.

At work, she has periodically shut the door to her office to consume large amounts of desserts, and she will not answer the phone or door while she is eating these foods. Ginger describes these times as being "like a fog" and denies that she is making the decision to eat the entire portion but rather says that the food is simply gone quickly. She denies the use of laxatives, compulsive exercise, or other attempts to undo the intake of sweets.

She reports that her episodes of binge eating occur 3–5 times weekly, and she cannot often predict when they will happen. While shopping for clothes this week, she stood in line to check out and purchased a large box of gift chocolates (approximately 40 pieces) and ate the entire box before arriving home. She stopped at a gas station to throw away the box and receipt before arriving home. After an incident like this, she describes feeling depressed, disgusted, discouraged, and hopeless. She also experiences increased cravings for sweets and carbohydrates following these episodes. She notes that the medications prescribed by her primary care provider have helped somewhat by reducing her appetite, but she adds, "I really don't need to be hungry to eat anyway." Past attempts at weight loss have included Weight Watchers, the Atkins diet, low-carbohydrate diets, Medifast, Slim Fast, calorie restriction, and over-the-counter supplements. None of these have been effective, per Ginger, because in the past year, she has not gone longer than 3 weeks without a binge episode.

She describes her marriage as a happy one and says that she and her husband are "entirely food focused." They both enjoy cooking, trying new recipes, watching cooking shows, eating out, and planning trips around meals. She loves pasta and potato dishes and notes that growing up in an Italian family, meals were often centered around numerous starchy carbohydrates. Her husband is also overweight, but she does not believe he secretly eats as she does. She has not shared with him her habit of eating secretly and eating large amounts of sweets at one sitting.

Ginger describes herself as friendly, a leader, and agreeable overall. Few people know when she is upset, she states, and she often withholds her emotions from colleagues, friends, and even close family. She equates anger with screaming and yelling, and she therefore would rather deal with a situation independently or ignore it in hopes of it resolving on its own. Despite her 22-year marriage to a man whom she describes as "compassionate and loving," she rarely expresses her displeasure with him, and oftentimes he does not know that she is upset about something. This is also true in her relationship with her two adult daughters. When situations arise at work that require her to advocate on behalf of her employees, she will do it but admits to significant anxiety and dread about being perceived as angry or unreasonable.

She speaks openly of the discrepancy between the success she has achieved in other areas of her life as a high-ranking hospital administrator, a mother, and wife and the lack of control she feels when it comes to food. She describes herself as a "complete failure" in regard to her eating and admits to feelings of significant low self-worth despite her success professionally and interpersonally. She has never received any treatment for her overeating and has never before seen a therapist. She has no prior inpatient or outpatient psychiatric history. She believes there have been times in her life when she has felt "pretty depressed," but she has never received any treatment, and these times gradually abated according to Ginger. She denies regular use of alcohol and drinks approximately one drink per month. She is negative for use of cocaine, marijuana, opioids, benzodiazepines, sedatives, hallucinogens, and other substances.

Ginger was raised in a small town in northern Michigan and is the youngest of three children. She has two older brothers and describes her childhood as "happy" overall, although she notes that she was the only "fat one" in the family and that this was often a source of ridicule from her mother, brothers, and peers at school. She believes weight first became an issue for her around the age of 5, and she can recall early memories of her mother scolding her for eating large portions. She recalls an incident around age 7 that involved her mother bringing home a large cake and setting it on the table. Ginger was excited to see the cake and asked her mother to try a piece. Apparently disturbed by Ginger's enthusiasm and desire for the cake, Ginger's mother used her hand to wipe all of the icing off the top, and while putting her hand in Ginger's face asked, "Why do you like this so much? It's all just fat and that's why you're fat." Shortly after this incident, Ginger began to identify food, and sweets in particular, as a source of shame and guilt. She began taking her allowance money and riding her bike to the corner store to purchase large amounts of chocolate, which she would eat in one sitting before heading home. She recalls that her mother questioned where her money was being spent but that no one ever knew about her secret eating. In front of friends and family, Ginger became very aware of the importance of limiting her portions and not eating seconds. She remembers some family members wondering why her weight was continuing to rise when she simply ate what all of the other members of her family were eating; they were not aware of her secret binge episodes. As she aged, the tension in her family on the topic of her weight continued to worsen, with her brothers often teasing her and peers at school ridiculing her. She had friends but few boyfriends and was not particularly physically active in her youth, preferring reading and schoolwork.

At age 22, she married her current husband and went on to have two daughters (now ages 30 and 27). She is close to them, although they both live several hours away. Her younger daughter "may also struggle with food"; she is overweight and very focused on food according to Ginger.

She remembers as a child hearing rumors that her mother had an eating disorder and describes her mother as very thin and a controlled eater. She also vaguely remembers hearing that her mother was institutionalized and received electroconvulsive therapy for a time before her marriage to Ginger's father, but this fact was never discussed at home nor was her mother's own relationship to food. Her mother passed away 6 months earlier at the age of 95.

See Video 1 for a role modeling of the clinical encounter between Ginger and her therapist. Note how the therapist elicits the different criteria for diagnosis of food addiction according to the YFAS and questions listed in Table 4–1. Be sure to pay particular attention to the relationship between food and mood for the patient and the role food plays in her current and past life

 Video Illustration 1: Diagnosing food addiction (7:06)

Discussion

Ginger is pleasant and cooperative during the interview and makes good eye contact. She processes easily and is often tearful, particularly when discussing the relationship she had with her mother. While she readily admits that her mother often used control and shame in relation to Ginger's food, she is reluctant to discuss any uncomfortable feelings associated with this and immediately follows up the stories of her childhood with "but she was a really good mom and a good woman." The guilt and shame that Ginger feels following an episode of binge eating (which are characteristic of persons with binge-eating disorder [BED]) appear to have originated in early childhood as she began to identify her eating and food desires as shameful and out of the ordinary, resulting in her hiding these behaviors.

She also is reluctant to discuss any hurt and anger she has toward her brothers, former classmates, current colleagues, or others, noting that anger serves "no purpose." When asked to elaborate on what anger looks like, she describes scenes from her childhood of fights between her parents that involved yelling, screaming, slamming doors, and dramatic exits from the home of one or both of her parents for a short time. She relays that she avoids these type of altercations at all costs and generally avoids the expression of negative feelings on the whole, as illustrated by her mentioning that her husband is rarely aware when she is upset or angry at him.

While the therapist gathers information from Ginger about her initiation of treatment, she expresses concern that Ginger may be addicted to food. Food addiction, although increasingly supported in the scientific literature in the fields of psychology and medicine, remains a hypothesis because it has not been declared a diagnosis in DSM-5 (American Psychiatric Association 2013). The YFAS is currently the most accurate measurement available to evaluate for food addiction (Gearhardt et al. 2009). This scale could be administered to determine if Ginger might be addicted to food.

Another disorder that would be high on the list of differential diagnoses for Ginger is BED. BED has been added to the list of feeding and eating disorders and generally describes many of the signs and symptoms we associate with the food addiction hypothesis and many symptoms we see in Ginger. It is important to note, however, that distinctions do exist between the two. In particular, one study suggested that as many as 24% of persons who met criteria for food addiction did not meet the criteria for BED (Davis et al. 2011). Similarly, those who meet criteria according to the YFAS often present with a more depressed affect, reduced emotion regulation, lower self-esteem, and higher prevalence of mood disorders compared with those with BED (Gearhardt et al. 2012). Ginger also denies purging, which helps to narrow the differential of eating disorders in her case.

Additionally, whereas Ginger is considered morbidly obese with a BMI of 47, it is important to note that not all obese individuals are addicted to food or have BED, nor are all persons with food addiction obese. Therefore, this distinction can be made only through a detailed workup of the patient. Food itself also can have different effects on different populations. This is because patients can adopt different styles of interacting with food that are referred to as *information gathering and sharing styles* (IGS). These styles can be translated into different stimulation or inhibition patterns of the same neurotransmitters, and therefore, an understanding of the individual's IGS style is critical to the successful treatment of disease (Shriner and Gold 2013).

To summarize, Ginger presents with the following: eating larger portions than most others would consider normal in a discreet period of time, a sense of lack of control over eating during the episode, eating more rapidly than normal, eating until uncomfortably full, eating large amounts of food when not feeling hungry, eating alone because of the embarrassment of how much one is eating, feeling disgusted after an episode of binge eating, marked distress surrounding the binge-eating episodes, binge eating not associated with any compensatory behavior (like purging or exercise), and binge eating occurring at least once a week for 3 months (in Ginger's case, the episodes have been occurring approximately 3–5 times weekly for at least 1 year). Although food addiction is a more novel hypothesis, the YFAS should be administered, and food addiction should be considered as a diagnosis in cases such as Ginger's.

Treatment

Because of the striking similarities in the brains and behaviors of persons with substance use disorders and those with food addiction, the approach to patient care has many areas of overlap. As is the case with other substance disorders, it is important for patients to be educated relative to the neurobiological and neurochemical aspects of food addiction. Patients should be counseled and taught about the new and exciting research in this field that has been conducted in the past several years; this research has shown the brains of obese persons and those with drug dependence to be strikingly similar. Most notably, the brains of these individuals were shown to have fewer dopamine receptors, and dopamine is the neurotransmitter most associated with pleasure and reward. While it is unclear if these persons were born with fewer receptors or if they were lost as a result of compulsive overeating, this may result in the person seeking greater quantities of highly palatable food to achieve the same brain reward as an individual with a normal amount of dopamine receptors (Smith and Robbins 2013). Educating the patient about food addiction, as we do in treatment for substance abuse, is thus the key for the patient to truly understand his or her disease.

Following education, as with other substance-related disorders, the 12-step model of recovery has been shown to assist those struggling with food addiction. Recovery groups such as Overeaters Anonymous (OA) and Food Addicts Anonymous (FAA) have increased in size and number over the years. These groups often view the associated addiction as a physical, mental, and spiritual condition that requires outside help and support from other members. Patients suspected of having BED or food addiction should be encouraged to attend OA or FAA meetings to establish a support network (Werdell 2009).

When treating addiction of any kind, the most important first step is to avoid continued use of the addicting substance. In the case of substance use disorders, patients are encouraged to abstain and/or enter a facility for detoxification. Because abstaining from all food is not possible for food addicts, they are instead encouraged to avoid the highly addictive foods such as sugar, flour, and salt because these can often serve as neurochemical triggers for binge episodes (Werdell 2009). Once they have secured a period of detox and abstinence, therapy to address the psychological and emotional causes and consequences of the addiction may commence.

There are many different therapeutic models to draw upon when treating Ginger and others like her. Psychodynamic theorists encourage the recognition and expression of feelings, particularly the negative feelings, as a means of achieving catharsis and eventually establishing new and more functional coping mechanisms. As is seen with Ginger, she has challenges when it comes to expressing her negative emotions, so much so that her husband, daughters, and coworkers are often unaware of her anger. Through mindfulness-based cognitive therapy, patients are encouraged to become aware of unresolved emotional suffering from childhood in addition to current patterns of behavior (Woolhouse et al. 2012). In subsequent therapy sessions, Ginger should be encouraged to call upon the feelings she experienced surrounding her eating as a young girl and to see what pattern she began to create around her eating in an attempt to avoid feeling her negative emotions. The goal would be for her to learn new ways of effectively identifying and expressing her thoughts and feelings. Also, by understanding her IGS and relationship with food, mindfulness can help her to start to change this relationship herself.

In addition to community resources, decreasing palatable food intake, and therapy, pharmacologic treatments are becoming more utilized. In the past, typical pharmacological treatments consisted of appetite suppressants for obese individuals. However, these treatments are largely ineffective for those with food addiction because these individuals do not generally report an association between hunger and the occurrence of a binge episode. In addition, the safety profiles and lack of overall efficacy of appetite suppressants have not made them ideal agents for use in this population. For food addiction, other pharmacological options have been made available for patients including lorcaserin (Belviq), a medication the U.S. Food and Drug Administration approved in 2010, which is believed to target serotonin 5-HT$_{2C}$ and cause satiety, and Qsymia (a combination of phentermine and Topamax) (Holes-Lewis et al. 2013). Ginger was prescribed Qsymia. While the combination of phentermine and Topamax can often assist in appetite and craving reduction, the medications have limited effectiveness in persons with food addiction, as is seen with Ginger. Additional pharmacotherapies are in the experimental phase in this population. A drug combination that is promising is the use of naltrexone plus baclofen, which causes weight loss by changing and reinforcing food preferences (Shriner and Gold 2013). Also, naltrexone combined with bupropion (a dopamine agonist) has been an effective anorexic drug, in which naltrexone blocks the μ opioid stimulus/reward aspects of food, while bupropion blocks appetitive desire (Shriner and Gold 2013).

Finally, bariatric surgery is often seen as an effective and available option to treat obese individuals with a BMI of greater than 40. However, because of the neurological, psychological, and emotional complexity of food addiction, this option and pharmacological options should never be used as a sole treatment option for food-addicted patients and should not be the first choice of physicians (Werdell 2009).

Conclusion

Changing behavior in all patients, but especially food-addicted patients, is challenging. While clinicians treating obesity often require monthly visits for the first 6 months to assist in behavior eradication and the development of new eating techniques, follow-up treatment for patients with food addiction likely requires even more frequent visits. Patients may need to be seen weekly or biweekly for the first several months of treatment.

Key Points

- Food addiction, like other addictions, is a disease with a neurobiological basis related to dopamine.

- The Yale Food Addiction Scale is the best clinical measure for food addiction and should be administered clinically to patients.

- Pharmacological treatment, in combination with therapy and reduction of palatable food intake, is effective in the population with food addiction.

References

American Psychiatric Association: Diagnostic and Statistical Manual of Mental Disorders, 5th Edition. Arlington, VA, American Psychiatric Association, 2013

Avena NM, Murray S, Gold MS: The next generation of obesity treatments: beyond suppressing appetite. Front Psychol 4:721, 2013 24130541

Davis C, Curtis C, Levitan RD, et al: Evidence that 'food addiction' is a valid phenotype of obesity. Appetite 57(3):711–717, 2011 21907742

Gearhardt AN, Corbin WR, Brownell KD: Preliminary validation of the Yale Food Addiction Scale. Appetite 52(2):430–436, 2009 19121351

Gearhardt AN, White MA, Masheb RM, et al: An examination of the food addiction construct in obese patients with binge eating disorder. Int J Eat Disord 45(5):657–663, 2012 22684991

Gold MS: From bedside to bench and back again: a 30-year saga. Physiol Behav 104(1):157–161, 2011 21530563

Holes-Lewis KA, Malcolm R, O'Neil PM: Pharmacotherapy of obesity: clinical treatments and considerations (Review). Am J Med Sci 345(4):284–288, 2013 23531960

Shriner RL, Gold MS: Is your patient addicted to food? Obesity Consults 1(1):8–10, 2013

Smith DG, Robbins TW: The neurobiological underpinnings of obesity and binge eating: a rationale for adopting the food addiction model. Biol Psychiatry 73(9):804–810, 2013 23098895

Werdell P: Bariatric Surgery and Food Addiction: Preoperative Considerations. Sarasota, FL, Evergreen Publications, 2009

Woolhouse H, Knowles A, Crafti N: Adding mindfulness to CBT programs for binge eating: a mixed-methods evaluation. Eat Disord 20(4):321–339, 2012 22703573

Questions

1.   If you have a patient and suspect that he or she might be a food addict, what is the best way to assess the patient's condition?

      A. Ask the patient if he or she feels addicted to food.
      B. Ask the patient if he or she can eat just one french fry.
      C. Ask the patient if he or she has a family history of addiction.
      D. Use the Yale Food Addiction Scale.

The correct answer is D.

The Yale Food Addiction Scale has been proven effective and predictive of disease in many populations. It is the first of its kind to measure food addiction and can aid diagnosticians in their differential diagnosis.

2.   What is the difference between binge-eating disorder (BED) and food addiction?

      A. Some food addicts have BED.
      B. Food addicts are more depressed and tend to have more mood disorders.
      C. BED is not in DSM-5.
      D. Food addiction is in DSM-5.

The correct answer is B.

As many as 24% of people who are addicted to food do not have BED. Typically, those who meet criteria for food addiction often have a more depressed affect, reduced emotion regulation, lower self-esteem, and higher prevalence of mood disorders compared with those with BED. BED does appear in DSM-5; food addiction does not.

3.   True or false: all obese people are addicted to food?

      A. True.
      B. False.

The correct answer is B.

Not all obese individuals are addicted to food, nor are all persons with food addiction obese.

CHAPTER 5

Gambling Disorder

Carla J. Rash, Ph.D.
Nancy M. Petry, Ph.D.

GAMBLING disorder refers to a pattern of gambling leading to negative consequences (e.g., financial, relationships, legal) that is difficult for a patient to control. This disorder affects between 0.4% and 4.0% of the general population in their lifetime and affected between 0.1% and 1.9% in the past year in North America (Petry 2005). Beyond those diagnosed with a gambling disorder, individuals with subclinical but still problematic gambling, called *problem gambling,* contribute an additional 1.3%–7.5% to the lifetime and 0.4%–3.6% to the past-year estimates. Gambling disorder is currently classified as a behavioral addiction under the "Substance-Related and Addictive Disorders" chapter of DSM-5 (American Psychiatric Association 2013). However, in DSM-III and DSM-IV (American Psychiatric Association 1980, 1994), it was categorized as an impulse-control disorder and had the label *pathological gambling disorder.* This move to the "Substance-Related and Addictive Disorders" chapter acknowledges the many similarities between gambling disorder and substance use disorders, although the criteria for gambling disorder have largely remained the same. Diagnosis of gambling disorder is given when clients meet four or more of the following: 1) often feels preoccupied with gambling, 2) needs to gamble in increasing amounts of money in order to achieve excitement, 3) makes repeated unsuccessful efforts to reduce or stop gambling, 4) experiences restlessness or irritability when trying to reduce or stop gambling, 5) gambles in response to negative moods, 6) chases loses, 7) lies to others to conceal the extent of gambling, 8) jeopardizes relationships, career, or educational opportunities because of gambling, and 9) relies on others to escape negative financial consequences of gambling (i.e., "bailouts").

In the following clinical case, we describe the case of Stanley, who exhibits some of the common features we encounter in treatment-seeking individuals with gambling disorder. He is a high-functioning professional whose gambling escalated beyond his control and led to some very serious negative consequences in his life. His treatment story typifies the ambivalence toward change that many individuals struggling with addictions, including gambling disorder, exhibit in a treatment setting.

Clinical Case

Stanley first sought individual counseling for problems related to anxiety. The 48-year-old, white, unmarried professional attributes the onset of his symptoms to financial stressors, including threat of bankruptcy and home foreclosure. He describes himself as "a worrier" for most of his adolescent and adult life, but he says that this trait had no significant negative impact on his life until the past 3 years. When the clinical history was taken by the initial therapist, it became evident that disordered gambling was a major contributor to the patient's current financial situation and related anxiety. Because the gambling was ongoing, the therapist referred Stanley for treatment specific to gambling.

At his initial visit for gambling treatment, Stanley reports frequent casino gambling (4–8 times per month). Despite a $150,000 annual salary, Stanley reports living paycheck to paycheck, often prioritizing gambling expenditures over living expenses. He hides the extent of his gambling from family and his significant other, lying about the reasons for his current financial status. He borrowed money from family several times to avoid foreclosure on his home.

Stanley first gambled in his early 20s via casino trips with friends. He maintained a nonproblematic pattern of moderate-frequency casino gambling within budgeted amounts for the next 10 years. In his early 30s, he experienced a substantial win ($100,000). Following this win, Stanley gambled more frequently and with larger sums of money. He often gambled in binges (e.g., 24–48 hours) with little to no sleep. These prolonged gambling episodes would impact his work, and he experienced significant stress during these periods. He gambled occasionally during the work week, usually after a major loss and in response to a desire to recoup losses.

Stanley gambled away his prior winnings. He began using his regular income and eventually accessed savings and retirement accounts to fund his gambling. Although aware that his gambling was excessive, he was convinced that another win was due to him and that such a win would rectify his problems. He periodically tried to limit gambling time and expenditures but repeatedly failed to adhere to his goals. As his financial situation deteriorated, he began to experience symptoms of anxiety, including excessive worry, difficulty concentrating, irritability, fatigue, and sleep disturbances. Gambling temporarily relieves these symptoms, providing hope that he might repair his finances quickly. Gambling losses worsen his symptoms, and these losses often trigger additional gambling episodes in an attempt to recoup money.

See Video 2 for an enactment of the introductory exchange between Stanley and the therapist. Note the role "chasing his losses" (a diagnostic criteria) plays in his gambling pattern and related consequences. In this initial vignette, Stanley mentions gambling as a strategy to make money and rectify his finances; this idea will be a major trigger for gambling urges during the early phase of treatment.

 Video Illustration 2: Introductory therapist-patient exchange (6:00)

Stanley has poor insight into the nature of his gambling disorder—he acknowledges that his gambling is out of control, but he also feels that a big win would solve all of his problems, including his anxiety, his financial difficulties, and the gambling problem itself. He focuses on his financial problems to the exclusion of other consequences of gambling, maintaining the belief that a "big win" would also solve other problems (i.e., eliminate the need to lie to family/ friends, improve anxiety and mood). He believes that he will be able to control his gambling easily once he resolves his financial problems, and he fails to recognize the maladaptive gambling patterns that have led to his current situation. In general, he attributes his financial losses to recent bad luck rather than a prolonged period of disordered gambling.

The patient exhibits several cognitive distortions common to problem gamblers, including 1) the gambler's fallacy (the belief that a string of losses must predict an imminent win), 2) availability heuristic (selective recall of wins over losses), 3) failure to recognize net losses that included some small wins (e.g., spending $400 and having a $50 win is deemed a success even though the net loss is $350), 4) the idea that his need to win will affect outcomes, and 5) beliefs about luck. These and other cognitions associated with gambling are described by Petry (2005).

In terms of treatment, he is ambivalent about abstaining from gambling. He acknowledges that continued gambling is worsening his circumstances, and he is willing to engage in treatment, but he is reluctant to give up what is, in his view, the only solution available to him. Given Stanley's inability to successfully control his gambling, the therapist recommends complete abstinence from gambling as a goal for treatment. Stanley is unwilling to commit to this goal, leading to a discussion of the benefits and risks of abstinence and controlled gambling goals. Stanley believes controlled gambling is a more realistic objective for him, and he and the therapist collaboratively define what *controlled gambling* would be for his situation and goals. For Stanley, these limits include no more than one casino trip per month and a limit of $100 per month for gambling activities. Although $100 may be a large gambling expenditure for some patients, it represents a substantial reduction from Stanley's current gambling habits. Stanley and the therapist agree to reevaluate the controlled gambling goal during treatment.

Stanley completes eight sessions of cognitive-behavioral treatment for pathological gambling as described by Petry (2005) and outlined in Table 5–1. Stanley greatly reduces his gambling frequency and intensity from baseline activity levels, but he gambles weekly and exceeds his self-defined limits for controlled gambling. After reviewing progress, the therapist opens a discussion regarding whether controlled gambling is a viable goal at this time. Stanley acknowledges that gambling episodes often trigger additional gambling and that once engaged in gambling he is unable to limit himself to predetermined monetary amounts. He recognizes that he is unable to control his gambling, and he agrees to a goal of complete abstinence from gambling during the remainder of his treatment period.

In addition, Stanley and the therapist discuss the potential barriers to meeting his therapeutic goals and whether these barriers can be addressed. Stanley identifies several key steps from his therapist's recommendations that he was reluctant to take in regard to his gambling. He decides to withdraw from the casino loyalty programs, whose e-mails and promotional contacts serve as triggers for gambling urges. He also agrees to join the self-exclusion program at his primary casinos. With these measures in place, the patient makes substantial progress during the remainder of treatment. He reports two casino gambling episodes in weeks 5–8, but he is successful in limiting the monetary amount. In discussing these lapses with his therapist, Stanley notes that he gambled in the hopes of quieting his gambling urges, but, instead, he experienced intensified urges following each episode.

Over the course of treatment, Stanley gains insight into his gambling behavior and cognitions. Financial stress is a key trigger for his gambling episodes, and his therapist encourages Stanley to seek financial counseling. Although directly addressing his financial problems is anxiety provoking, Stanley finds that he is better able to control his worry and anxiety when he develops a concrete financial plan and begins working toward these goals. He is also encouraged to complement his individual therapy by attending self-help Gamblers Anonymous (GA) group meetings.

Discussion

Stanley experienced a major win that precipitated the development of his gambling disorder. Prior to this win, he gambled regularly but was consistently able to stay within his planned expenditure goal and did not exhibit other problematic behaviors related to gambling (e.g., chasing losses, gambling in response to emotions). The availability of winnings permitted Stanley to use larger sums of money during gambling episodes, which escalated the excitement he experienced. As his winnings disappeared, smaller gambling expenditures were not sufficient to achieve these levels of excitement, and he continued to gamble with larger amounts than his finances could support. In our clinical experience, many disordered gamblers describe an early win (albeit most often not as large as Stanley's win) that leads to increased gambling frequency and expenditure. These wins, even if they are only $100–$500 in magnitude, can increase the excitement about gambling (akin to the high of addictions) and may also distort perceptions of gambling skill and/or expected returns from gambling, as well as strengthen irrational beliefs about gambling (e.g., illusion of control). However, we note that although early or major wins are common among problem gamblers and may be a risk factor for the development of problems in some gamblers (Turner et al. 2006), these wins are not necessary for the development or diagnosis of gambling disorder.

TABLE 5–1.	Petry's (2005) cognitive-behavioral treatment for gambling disorder
Session 1	The first session focuses on increasing patients' recognition of gambling triggers, including the cues (e.g., cash), events (e.g., celebrations, arguments), days/times, people, and emotions (e.g., negative affect) that precipitate gambling episodes.
Session 2	Building on session 1, patients learn to examine their gambling episodes using a functional analysis. Antecedents and negative and positive consequences of each gambling episode are considered.
Session 3	Increasing alternate pleasurable activities is the focus. Some patients may return to hobbies or activities popular from their past. Others may pursue new interests. Possible activities should span a range, including those that require planning and those that can be done spur of the moment. Both solo and social activities should be included; attention to costs of activities and inclusion of some activities that are low- or no-cost are important.
Session 4	This session focuses on managing triggers, including anticipating future triggers (e.g., payday) and making plans for how to avoid or cope with both anticipated and unanticipated triggers.
Session 5	Patients learn relaxation techniques to manage responses to gambling urges.
Session 6	The content of this session focuses on handling interpersonal conflicts, including practicing gambling refusal skills.
Session 7	This session addresses the common cognitive biases and distortions experienced by those with gambling disorder.
Session 8	The last session focuses on relapse prevention, with emphasis on major life events that could precipitate a relapse to gambling (e.g., retirement, divorce, death of family member).

Stanley is also rather typical in regard to his poor insight into his gambling problem. His initial choice to seek treatment for anxiety rather than gambling may be an example of this poor insight, but it could also be related to the stigma of seeking treatment for addictions, including behavioral addictions such as gambling. In addition, many gamblers perceive disordered gambling to be a problem of limited finances. That is, if they only had more money, they would not have a gambling problem, and this belief may also impede seeking treatment. Disordered gamblers often fail to recognize the pattern of behavior that resulted in their current situation and believe that more of the same behavior will produce different results. They often believe they are in control or can easily regain control of their gambling. In many cases, it is only with repeated failures to stop or cut down their gambling that patients begin to perceive their behavior as problematic or uncontrollable and consider the possibility of seeking treatment. Often, the problem gambler has been encouraged to seek treatment by family, friends, financial advisors or debt management counselors, lawyers, or other therapists.

In the "Assessment" section, we discuss some features relevant to Stanley's diagnosis and treatment planning.

Assessment

A thorough assessment of gambling criteria and behavior can be useful not only for diagnosis but also for providing personalized feedback to the patient. This feedback on his or her gambling often represents the patient's first attempt to see his or her own gambling behavior from a more objective perspective.

Several structured clinical interviews are available to identify and assess the DSM-5 symptoms of gambling disorder. The National Opinion Research Center DSM-IV Screen for Gambling Problems (Gerstein et al. 1999) assesses lifetime and past-year gambling criteria, with scores of 5 or greater indicating pathological gambling. Stanley scored 7 out of 10 possible on this measure, endorsing the following items: preoccupation with gambling, escalating gambling to achieve desired excitement, unsuccessful attempts to control gambling, gambling as an emotional escape or way of coping, chasing losses, lying to family and friends to conceal extent of gambling, and asking for bailouts.

Stanley also completed the Gambling Timeline Followback (Weinstock et al. 2004) for gambling in the past 30 days prior to his intake appointment. These baseline estimates of gambling frequency and expenditure were useful for providing psychoeducation to Stanley, particularly in comparing the severity of his gambling to recreational and nonproblem gambling patterns. Ongoing monitoring of gambling behavior using the Gambling Timeline Followback can also be helpful in evaluating treatment progress. Stanley reported four weekend casino trips with one additional nonweekend trip in the past month to chase his losses. Casino expenditures ranged from $600 to $2,400, with time spent between 2 and 12 hours per trip. In addition to discussing his gambling days (e.g., precipitants, ability to limit expenditures on some days but not others), the therapist also queried nongambling patterns. In particular, although Stanley chased his losses with a weekday trip to the casino once in the past month, he was able to inhibit this urge on other weeks. Stanley noted that larger losses created greater urges to return to the casino and that he was better able to deal successfully with these urges when he had social or work-related obligations that prevented him from going to the casino.

Assessment of activities on nongambling days can be also useful in determining whether patients have other pleasurable activities in their lives, which may be useful for treatment planning. In Stanley's case, he had relatively few alternate activities in his life, suggesting that building more pleasurable and planned activities may be an important treatment component for this patient. He could control his gambling to attend planned social events with his girlfriend or family. Increasing these activities, especially at high-risk times (e.g., at the end of a big work project), may help Stanley learn to manage gambling urges without gambling.

Differential Diagnoses

Mood and anxiety disorders, as well as substance use, have high comorbidity with gambling disorder (Petry et al. 2005). Clinicians may wish to evaluate for manic or hypomanic episodes, particularly if gambling activities increase suddenly in frequency or intensity (i.e., excessive involvement in pleasurable activities). In Stanley's case, his gambling remained at a fairly high and steady frequency. Although he reported elevated and expansive moods ("feeling on top of the world when winning," "like nothing could stop me"), these periods were limited to winning streaks. Evaluation should also include assessment of depressed mood and current and past suicide ideation and attempts. Whether because of the gambling disorder itself or the frequency of other comorbid disorders, rates of suicide ideation and suicide attempts are higher among disordered gamblers compared with the general population and may be related to gambling severity (Petry 2005).

Stanley experienced a number of symptoms related to generalized anxiety disorder, including excessive worry, for the past 3 years. Initially, the focus of his worry was confined to his financial circumstances; however, his anxiety extended to multiple domains over time, including work, health, and relationships. Stanley met criteria for both gambling disorder and generalized anxiety disorder.

Stanley reported no history of illicit substance use, and he did not meet criteria for alcohol use disorder. However, his alcohol use was closely tied with his casino gambling and occasionally exceeded at-risk levels (i.e., more than 4 drinks per episode or more than 14 drinks per week for men). Alcohol use, especially among risky drinkers, tends to decrease during gambling treatment (Rash et al. 2011). However, monitoring of his alcohol intake over the course of treatment is warranted.

Determinants

Another major factor in Stanley's difficulty limiting his gambling involved the casino loyalty programs. He was unwilling to forfeit these perks and would plan casino visits with the intention to only gamble a specified small amount of money in order to take advantage of the loyalty program offerings; however, he usually failed to stay within his budgeted amount once he began gambling. These loyalty perks and associated e-mails functioned as powerful and frequent triggers for gambling urges. At the beginning of treatment, his therapist recommended withdrawing from the loyalty programs; however, Stanley, like many other treatment-seeking gamblers, struggled with this decision. These occasions present an opportunity for a potentially therapeutic discussion that may include challenging the patient's beliefs about his ability to control his gambling. Stanley described a recent casino trip to take advantage of free tickets to a show. He intended to attend the show and leave without gambling. However, he was unable to resist the temptation to gamble and lost $750. After further discussion, Stanley began to see that this outcome was not an isolated event but was rather typical of his experiences, and he then made the decision to withdraw from the programs.

Negative affect was a major antecedent for Stanley. He gambled often to escape feelings of anxiety, and he enjoyed the temporary reprieve offered by planning or engaging in gambling. The functional analysis activities during treatment were useful in helping Stanley recognize that his behavior was part of a negative spiral. He gambled to relieve anxiety about his finances. Although gambling provided temporary relief, the usual consequence following the gambling episode was greater debt, leading to self-recrimination and heightened anxiety, which often triggered renewed desire to gamble.

In the "Treatment" section, we review treatment options available to patients with gambling disorder. Many states have helpline numbers available for individuals experiencing gambling problems. These numbers are often posted in casinos and advertised in general media outlets. The National Council on Problem Gambling maintains a 24-hour, confidential national helpline, and their Web site (www.ncpgambling.org) provides access to state-level resources related to problem gambling treatment. These resources can facilitate access to treatments that are available in the patient's community.

Treatment

Several treatments are available for problem gambling. Here, we briefly discuss GA and other self-help approaches, cognitive and cognitive-behavioral treatments, and brief motivational interventions. Last, we review briefly the pharmacotherapy options that have been evaluated in research trials.

GA group meetings are the most widely available treatment option and can be used alone or in conjunction with other interventions. GA is based on the 12-step approach of Alcoholics Anonymous, and groups are peer led and abstinence-focused. Individuals who engage in GA in conjunction with professional treatment have better outcomes than those who receive professional care but do not attend GA meetings (Petry 2003), but these improvements may be reflective of self-selection biases because the patients who supplement their professional treatment with GA may be more motivated to stop their gambling overall. Patients can find local groups online. In general, we recommend GA to all patients and provide a list of local GA group meetings at the first treatment session. Even for those patients who do not attend while they are receiving professional treatment, GA is a valuable resource in the event that gambling problems resurface in the future. Some GA meetings welcome family and friends to attend "open meetings," recognizing that the affects of problem gambling often extend far beyond the identified patient and that support from these individuals may be integral to the patient's recovery.

Self-help treatments have the advantage of reducing barriers to treatment, including cost, transportation, child care needs, and stigma. Bibliotherapy and self-directed Internet interventions are effective in reducing gambling compared with wait list control groups in a number of studies (e.g., Labrie et al. 2012). Many disordered gamblers may prefer these self-help options as a first-treatment option, and for some, this intervention may help them successfully reduce their gambling.

Cognitive-behavioral therapy (CBT) focuses on changing both cognitions and behaviors related to gambling. Petry's (2005) eight-session format is outlined in Table 5–1. CBT is effective compared with GA-only comparison conditions and therapist-delivered, as opposed to patient-directed (i.e., workbooks), strategies; CBT results in increased engagement and improved outcomes (Petry et al. 2006). Brief four- to six-session CBT interventions also show some promise with problem and pathological gambling of college students (Larimer et al. 2012), but further evaluation of this intervention is needed in broader samples of treatment-seeking gamblers.

Cognitive interventions that focus on the maladaptive thought processes involved in gambling are also available. These therapies assume that cognitive distortions about gambling play a key role in the development of gambling disorder and that correction of these beliefs will lead to more logical choices in behavior—ultimately, reduction in or abstention from gambling. Ladouceur et al.'s (2001) intervention provides weekly sessions until the patient stops gambling, up to maximum of 20 sessions. Session content addresses identification and correction of common cognitive distortions among gamblers. The second therapy component is relapse prevention, which involves identification of high-risk situations for relapse and maladaptive beliefs related to gambling control. Short-term outcomes improved among patients receiving cognitive therapy relative to wait list control groups (Ladouceur et al. 2001).

Brief motivational interventions have also shown promise for reducing gambling, either delivered alone or in conjunction with professionally delivered or self-help (e.g., workbooks) therapies. Often, these interventions have been directed at individuals with subclinical diagnoses—those who do not meet criteria for gambling disorder but experience negative consequences related to gambling. These interventions may also be useful for engaging individuals, like Stanley, who have poor problem recognition, in further treatment or for spurring self-directed change. Session content generally includes personalized feedback, brief advice, review of options (e.g., treatment options, change goals), and self-efficacy building, all delivered in an empathic manner. A brief motivational telephone intervention combined with a self-help workbook was effective in improving gambling outcomes in problem gamblers (e.g., Hodgins et al. 2001). Single-session stand-alone motivational sessions have also been effective compared with an assessment-only control group (e.g., Larimer et al. 2012). Direct comparisons of motivational and CBT approaches suggest both interventions are equally effective relative to control comparisons in problem gamblers (e.g., Petry et al. 2009).

Currently, no pharmacotherapies are approved for the treatment of gambling disorder in the United States, and only a limited number of trials have evaluated potential medications for this purpose. These trials have focused on opioid antagonists, selective serotonin and norepinephrine/dopamine reuptake inhibitors, and mood stabilizers. More research is needed to evaluate efficacy and adverse effects in this population before medications can be recommended as a first-line option for the treatment of gambling disorder. However, providers may find that medications to treat comorbid disorders are necessary (Petry 2005), and such treatment may ease symptoms to an extent that the patient can engage more fully in gambling treatment.

Conclusion

The clinical case illustrated here presents several common issues prevalent among those seeking treatment, including the presence of comorbid disorders, cognitive distortions about gambling, ambivalence about abstaining from gambling, and difficulty taking concrete steps to reduce gambling during treatment. Gambling disorder can result in substantial negative consequences for patients and their families. Fortunately, several treatment options are available, ranging from self-help to brief inventions to intensive therapies. These treatments are efficacious in reducing gambling problems and provide choices for patients with differing needs and concerns.

Key Points

- Gambling disorder affects about 1%–2% of individuals in the United States throughout their lifetime.

- Individuals with gambling problems can experience many negative consequences as a result of their gambling, including mental health, financial, legal, and family relationship issues.

- Gambling disorder has high comorbidity rates with anxiety, mood, and substance use disorders.

- A variety of effective treatment options are available, including self-help, cognitive and cognitive-behavioral treatments, and brief motivational interventions.

References

American Psychiatric Association: Diagnostic and Statistical Manual of Mental Disorders, 3rd Edition. Washington, DC, American Psychiatric Association, 1980

American Psychiatric Association: Diagnostic and Statistical Manual of Mental Disorders, 4th Edition. Washington, DC, American Psychiatric Association, 1994

American Psychiatric Association: Diagnostic and Statistical Manual of Mental Disorders, 5th Edition. Arlington, VA, American Psychiatric Publishing, 2013

Gerstein D, Hoffman J, Larison C, et al: Gambling Impact and Behavior Study: Report to the National Gambling Impact Study Commission. Chicago, IL, National Opinion Research Center at the University of Chicago, 1999

Hodgins DC, Currie SR, el-Guebaly N: Motivational enhancement and self-help treatments for problem gambling. J Consult Clin Psychol 69(1):50–57, 2001 11302277

Labrie RA, Peller AJ, Laplante DA, et al: A brief self-help toolkit intervention for gambling problems: a randomized multisite trial. Am J Orthopsychiatry 82(2):278–289, 2012 22506530

Ladouceur R, Sylvain C, Boutin C, et al: Cognitive treatment of pathological gambling. J Nerv Ment Dis 189(11):774–780, 2001 11758661

Larimer ME, Neighbors C, Lostutter TW, et al: Brief motivational feedback and cognitive behavioral interventions for prevention of disordered gambling: a randomized clinical trial. Addiction 107(6):1148–1158, 2012 22188239

Petry NM: Patterns and correlates of Gamblers Anonymous attendance in pathological gamblers seeking professional treatment. Addict Behav 28(6):1049–1062, 2003 12834650

Petry NM: Pathological Gambling: Etiology, Comorbidity, and Treatment. Washington, DC, American Psychological Association, 2005

Petry NM, Stinson FS, Grant BF: Comorbidity of DSM-IV pathological gambling and other psychiatric disorders: results from the National Epidemiologic Survey on Alcohol and Related Conditions. J Clin Psychiatry 66(5):564–574, 2005 15889941

Petry NM, Ammerman Y, Bohl J, et al: Cognitive-behavioral therapy for pathological gamblers. J Consult Clin Psychol 74(3):555–567, 2006 16822112

Petry NM, Weinstock J, Morasco BJ, et al: Brief motivational interventions for college student problem gamblers. Addiction 104(9):1569–1578, 2009 19686527

Rash CJ, Weinstock J, Petry NM: Drinking patterns of pathological gamblers before, during, and after gambling treatment. Psychol Addict Behav 25(4):664–674, 2011 21928867

Turner N, Zangeneh M, Littman-Sharp N: The experience of gambling and its role in problem gambling. International Gambling Studies 6:237–266, 2006

Weinstock J, Whelan JP, Meyers AW: Behavioral assessment of gambling: an application of the timeline followback method. Psychol Assess 16(1):72–80, 2004 15023094

Questions

1.   Gambling disorder is classified under which category in DSM-5?

   A. Disruptive, impulse control, and conduct disorders.
   B. Adjustment disorders.
   C. Substance-related and addictive disorders.
   D. Neurocognitive disorders.

   The correct answer is C.

   Gambling disorder is classified under the substance-related and addictive disorders section as the only behavioral addiction in DSM-5. In DSM-III and DSM-IV, gambling was classified under impulse-control disorders.

2.   The behavior of those diagnosed with gambling disorder was given the label _____ in the DSM-III and DSM-IV systems.

   A. Pathological gambling.
   B. Problem gambling.
   C. Addicted gambling.
   D. Recreational gambling.

   The correct answer is A.

   This term was changed to gambling disorder in DSM-5. *Problem gambling* generally refers to subclinical, but still problematic, levels of gambling (i.e., those meeting two or three gambling criteria). Recreational and nonproblem gamblers are able to control their gambling and have not experienced significant negative consequences related to their gambling.

3.   Which of the following disorders is commonly comorbid with gambling disorder?

    A. Mood disorders.
    B. Anxiety disorders.
    C. Substance use disorders.
    D. All of the above.

The correct answer is D.

Prevalence of all of these disorders is elevated among those with gambling disorder relative to the general population.

CHAPTER 6

Internet Gaming Disorder

Virtual or Real?

Tolga Taneli, M.D.
Yu-Heng Guo, M.D.
Sabina Mushtaq, M.D.

ON October 18, 1958, visitors to the Brookhaven National Laboratory waited in line to play arguably the "first video game"—*Tennis for Two*—created by nuclear physicist William Higinbotham, head of the laboratory's Instrumentation Division. Hoping to "liven up the place to have a game that people could play…" during the annual visitors' day, Higinbotham connected an analog computer to an oscilloscope, giving visitors control of a moving dot between two invisible racquets controlled by buttons and dials (Brookhaven National Laboratory 2014). Perhaps more from novelty than the compulsion to play, long lines were said to have formed for a turn at the game.

Dr. Ivan K. Goldberg's 1995 tongue-in-cheek post, "Internet Addictive Disorder Diagnostic Criteria," on his Web site Depression Central was modeled after other addictive disorders in DSM-IV (American Psychiatric Association 1994) and included humorous references to "a great deal of time spent in activities related to Internet use (e.g., buying Internet books, trying out new WWW browsers, researching Internet vendors, organizing files of downloaded materials)" and "voluntary or involuntary typing movements of the fingers." He proposed tolerance and withdrawal symptoms for his fictitious disorder, but surprisingly, his well-subscribed Web site soon drew serious commenters who were experiencing those very symptoms (Goldberg 1995).

One of the earliest references to pathological gaming, as opposed to problematic Internet use, predates Goldberg. In his case report titled "Pathological

Preoccupation With Video Games," Keepers (1990) described the case of a pre-adolescent who had stolen, forged checks, and skipped school to continue using video games, albeit, not necessarily Internet games. The term *video game* represents a broad category of electronic games, not all of which are dependent on an Internet connection or interaction with other players. An industry report commissioned by the Entertainment Software Association (2013) claimed that 58% of Americans play video games, with 51% of U.S. households owning a dedicated game console and 36% of gamers playing on their smartphones. About a third of players are under 18 years of age. Another third are between 18 and 35; the remaining third are older than 36 years of age. The average player is 30 years old. Women make up 45% of the gaming population. The most common online games are puzzles, board games, game shows, trivia, and card games. Although massively multiplayer online role-playing games (MMORPGs; see Table 6–1) are not the most common type of online game, they represent the bulk of the discussion in publications concerned with Internet gaming.

Early MMORPGs were modeled after their tabletop counterparts, such as the 1974 game *Dungeons & Dragons,* a fantasy role-playing game played, not unlike a traditional board game, on a gridded surface using polyhedral dice and involving storytelling over several play sessions. Current MMORPGs involve computer servers on several continents, engaging thousands of players at a time in fantasy story lines and battles. From humble beginnings, gaming has grown into a 15-billion-dollar-a-year industry. Just in the past decade, mobile devices have been added to the means of access, making gaming perpetually available.

Responding to criticism regarding the absence of age and content ratings similar to movies, the Entertainment Software Association established the Entertainment Software Rating Board, a nonprofit self-regulatory body, in 1994. The Entertainment Software Association reports that the rating system has been well received by players and parents. Yet the rating system offers no solace to excessive users, whose suffering became evident to researchers in the 1980s and 1990s, drawing immediate comparisons with other forms of behavioral addictions, including pathological gambling and excessive television viewing (Keepers 1990).

At its 2006 annual meeting, the American Medical Association (AMA) adopted Resolution 421 (A-05) (American Medical Association Council on Science and Public Health 2007), which asked "AMA's Council on Science and Public Health to work in conjunction with all appropriate specialty societies to prepare a report reviewing and summarizing the research data on the emotional and behavioral effects, including addiction potential, of video games" (p. 1). The council recommended that its final Report 12-A-07 be forwarded "to the American Psychiatric Association and other appropriate medical specialty societies for review and consideration in conjunction with the upcoming revision of the *Diagnostic and Statistical Manual of Mental Disorders*" (p. 10). The council also

TABLE 6–1.   Internet gaming glossary

Avatar	A virtual representation of oneself, whether as a character in a computer game or as an alias in an Internet forum.
Clans (also guilds)	An officially organized team of players that can play other teams. Members can be known as "clanners."
Console games	Games on dedicated gaming machines such as Nintendo, Sega, Xbox, and PlayStation—not to be confused with personal computer games.
First-person shooter (FPS)	A first-person weapon-based combat game with a cursor on the screen used to aim to kill opponents. Popular themes include historical wars, fighting aliens, and killing zombies—includes games such as *Call of Duty* (COD), *Counter-Strike,* and *Halo.*
Massively multiplayer online role-playing game (MMORPG), massively multiplayer online game (MMOG), persistent multiplayer universe game	A game where one creates an avatar in a virtual fantasy world and interacts with other online players to complete missions and journeys—including *World of Warcraft, RuneScape, Final Fantasy,* and, more recently, *Minecraft.* All avatars are part of the same persistent virtual world that continues to exist and change even when the player is off-line.
Persistent multiplayer universe games	See MMORPGs.
Person versus person (PvP)	In certain games, playing against another online gamer, as opposed to a nonplayer character controlled by the gaming application.
Real-time strategy (RTS)	An online strategy game, usually a war game, in which players mine for resources to produce units and structures to strategically conquer an opponent—includes *Starcraft* and *Command and Conquer.*
Third-person shooter (TPS)	A shooter game in which the player's character can be seen (e.g., *Tomb Raider*).

Source.   Some definitions are adapted from the following Web site: http://opencontent.org/wiki/index.php?title=Glossary_of_Gaming_Terms (Creative Commons Attribution 3.0 License, http://creativecommons.org/licenses/by/3.0/legalcode).

advocated that research into the effects of video games be funded by agencies such as the Centers for Disease Control and Prevention and National Institutes of Health.

The DSM-5 (American Psychiatric Association 2013) Task Force asked the 14-member Substance-Related Disorders Work Group to consider behavioral addictions, including gambling, Internet gaming, Internet use generally, work, shopping, and exercise. Not without controversy, the work group voted to move gambling disorder to the "Substance-Related and Addictive Disorders" section of DSM-5 and to include only one other condition—Internet gaming disorder (in Section III, "Emerging Measures and Models"). The decision was based on the large body of research and cases of documented severe consequences. The work group concluded that research on other behavioral addictions was relatively limited, and adverse consequences were less well documented.

While extensive, the research on Internet gaming did not apply standard diagnostic criteria; some reports used criteria paralleling those for substance use disorders and others borrowed from impulse control or pathological gambling criteria. DSM-5 now includes proposed criteria for Internet gaming disorder (see Box 6–1), with the hope of standardizing emerging work in the field. The description of criteria is adapted from a study in China (Tao et al. 2010) and includes references to withdrawal, tolerance, and failure to control gaming to the detriment of function.

Box 6–1. Proposed Criteria for Internet Gaming Disorder

Persistent and recurrent use of the Internet to engage in games, often with other players, leading to clinically significant impairment or distress as indicated by five (or more) of the following in a 12-month period:

1. Preoccupation with Internet games. (The individual thinks about previous gaming activity or anticipates playing the next game; Internet gaming becomes the dominant activity in daily life).
   Note: This disorder is distinct from Internet gambling, which is included under gambling disorder.
2. Withdrawal symptoms when Internet gaming is taken away. (These symptoms are typically described as irritability, anxiety, or sadness, but there are no physical signs of pharmacological withdrawal.)
3. Tolerance—the need to spend increasing amounts of time engaged in Internet games.
4. Unsuccessful attempts to control the participation in Internet games.
5. Loss of interests in previous hobbies and entertainment as a result of, and with the exception of, Internet games.
6. Continued excessive use of Internet games despite knowledge of psychosocial problems.
7. Has deceived family members, therapists, or others regarding the amount of Internet gaming.
8. Use of Internet games to escape or relieve a negative mood (e.g., feelings of helplessness, guilt, anxiety).

9. Has jeopardized or lost a significant relationship, job, or educational or career opportunity because of participation in Internet games.

Note: Only nongambling Internet games are included in this disorder. Use of the Internet for required activities in a business or profession is not included; nor is the disorder intended to include other recreational or social Internet use. Similarly, sexual Internet sites are excluded.

Specify current severity:

Internet gaming disorder can be mild, moderate, or severe depending on the degree of disruption of normal activities. Individuals with less severe Internet gaming disorder may exhibit fewer symptoms and less disruption of their lives. Those with severe Internet gaming disorder will have more hours spent on the computer and more severe loss of relationships or career or school opportunities.

Source.   Reprinted from the *Diagnostic and Statistical Manual of Mental Disorders,* 5th Edition. Arlington, VA, American Psychiatric Association, 2013. Used with permission. Copyright © 2013 American Psychiatric Association.

Clinical Case

James was always a bright student. His Korean parents fostered his education, perhaps at times excessively. Without effort, he was on the honor roll through high school. Now a freshman in college, he was going to sleep at odd hours, beginning his online time innocently enough "to check e-mail" and ending up playing *World of Warcraft*, an MMORPG, into the early morning hours—to the detriment of morning classes. When his parents proudly inquired about his grades during winter break, they were surprised to find out that he had mustered only mediocre grades. He reluctantly revealed this out of concern that he might lose his scholarship. This was not James' first time running into trouble with computer gaming. Although he had been on the soccer team in middle school, he was quick to get bored in high school and was regarded by his teacher as "not trying hard enough." He did not naturally make friends, preferring solitude. Throughout his senior year in high school, he spent progressively more time on the computer, dismissing his parents' attempts to engage him in family life, so he could "complete a mission with [his] clan and upgrade [his] avatar." Before the end of his senior year, his parents heeded the advice of the school social worker and took James to a child and adolescent psychiatrist whom he recommended. She diagnosed James with social anxiety disorder, also recognizing his excessive time spent gaming. Whether because of the individual sessions, the escitalopram that was prescribed for his anxiety, or the family sessions focusing on curbing his access to computers, James initially kept up with his schoolwork. Soon, though, he was skipping school, heading to Internet cafés to circumvent the move of his computer from his room to his parents' room. Not ready to give up, his parents enrolled James in "Rehab After School," a group therapy program for chemically addicted high school students. James was one of two in the group with Internet gaming problems. He eventually joined a church basketball team and was able to finish his senior year, staying away from Internet games for the entire second semester.

Away in college and without the watchful eyes of his parents, James drifted back to *World of Warcraft,* playing as many as 60 hours a week. James was not surprised by his midterm grades. Most nights he did not go to bed until the early morning hours, attending only evening classes. He began skipping cafeteria meals, opting for unhealthy snacks, because he was often "in the middle of an intense quest." He probably lost 10 pounds, he surmised. If it weren't for his parents' insistence, James was prepared not to go back home during the few short school breaks, preferring instead to stay in the dormitory. He, nevertheless, came home but made a point of planning his days there around his games. Seeing his preoccupation, his parents demanded some of his brief time at home, but they were met with anger and irritability. Their son once again was consumed by online games. James' parents stopped his gaming subscription payment. When James attempted to surreptitiously reactivate his payments on his father's credit card, his father punished him by cutting basic cable and Internet service to the house, which brought James to the verge of physical confrontation.

When his psychiatrist sees him after a hiatus, she finds him to be underweight and tired, if not also somewhat depressed. Speaking into his lap, he describes his mood as "okay." While not overtly sad, he fails to brighten much. He has little rationale to explain his excessive gaming, other than to comment: "I am really good at *World of Warcraft,* but if I don't keep up, people will catch up to me!" The psychiatrist ascertains that James has not been using drugs or alcohol in college and that his Internet addiction does not involve pornography or gambling.

James has continued taking escitalopram since starting college. He also agrees to individual therapy at the college's student health clinic, but his attendance there is sporadic. Because of his failing grades, and at the behest of his parents, counselor, and psychiatrist, James decides to take a term off from school and attend an inpatient Internet addiction program.

See Video 3 for a dramatization of a typical encounter with a patient with Internet gaming disorder. Note how the doctor establishes rapport with the patient by asking about what specific games he plays and using lingo such as "avatar." Pay close attention to how the doctor elicits the criteria for Internet gaming disorder during the encounter. Also, note how the doctor does a good job of screening for other associated behavioral addictions that are associated with the Internet, such as gambling and sex addictions.

 Video Illustration 3: Establishing rapport and assessing for Internet gaming disorder (4:46)

Discussion

"My child is on his phone/tablet/computer too much" is a ubiquitous concern for parents in industrialized countries. When is use problematic or even pathological? A broad range of studies, more than 250 of which were reviewed by the Substance-Related Disorders Work Group for the DSM-5 revision, have attempted to answer this question as it relates to Internet gaming. Whereas a uniform criteria set does not exist, many studies—and ultimately the proposed DSM-5 criteria set—were inspired by criteria for substance use disorders and pathological gambling. A uniform bar for impairment has also been absent, resulting in prevalence estimates among gamers from less than 1% to about 9%. Researchers have offered a number of assessment instruments, first to assess problematic Internet use and then, more specifically, Internet gaming addiction (see Table 6–2).

The Substance-Related Disorders Work Group concluded that there were many parallels among the addictive disorders under its purview for this most recent revision and Internet gaming disorder. In addition to describing withdrawal and tolerance symptoms, they identified preoccupation with gaming, attempts to reduce/stop, continued use despite problems, deception of others about use, escaping of adverse moods, and the loss (or risk of loss) of meaningful relationships and opportunities as hallmark features. Petry et al. (2014) provided a comprehensive review of the rationale for including Internet gaming disorder—but not the more global Internet addiction—in DSM-5. Translations of the consensus document into the 11 main languages of countries in which research on the condition has been most abundantly conducted (English, Spanish, Portuguese, Italian, French, German, Dutch, Turkish, Chinese, Korean, and Japanese) can be found online (www.niira.org.au/sites/default/files/an-international-consensus.pdf) as Appendix S1 of Petry et al. (2014).

As in James' case, attempts to evade curbs on use, including by deception, are not uncommon. Corroborative interviews with, for example, family members are mandatory and should verify time spent gaming as well as extent of impairment. A candid interview should elicit many of the symptoms from the patient (see Table 6–3).

The extent of traits or comorbid psychopathology has not been well defined or exhaustively studied. Nevertheless, some correlations have been observed in problematic gamers, including positive correlations for low self-esteem, depression, drinking, and conduct problems and a negative correlation for academic performance. Other authors have suggested higher prevalence rates of obsessive-compulsive disorder, generalized and social anxiety, attention-deficit/hyperactivity disorder, hypomania, obsessive-compulsive personality disorder, borderline personality disorder, avoidant personality disorder, and psychosis among Internet-addicted youth. The impairment of social interaction has also been well described. Bona fide mental disorders should be well explored, particularly depression, social anxiety, obsessive-compulsive disorder, and attention-deficit/hyperactivity disorder.

James is not unusual in his preoccupation with game play and his evasion of possible obstacles. Problem games appear frequently to aim to alter a negative

---

TABLE 6–2.   **Some assessment instruments for online gaming and Internet use**

Gaming-specific instruments

Game Addiction Scale (GAS)

Motives for Online Gaming Questionnaire (MOGQ)

Pathological Video Game Use (PVGU)

Problematic Online Gaming Questionnaire (POGQ)

Problematic Online Gaming Questionnaire–Short Form (POGQ-SF)

Video Game Addiction Scale (VGAS)

Video Game Dependency Scale–II (KFN-CSAS-II)

General Internet use instruments

Chinese Internet Addiction Inventory (CIAI)

Compulsive Internet Use Scale (CIUS)

Internet Related Problem Scale (IRPS)

Internet-Related Addictive Behavior Inventory (IRABI)

Nichols Internet Addiction Scale (NIAS)

Online Cognition Scale (OCS)

Problematic Internet Use Scale

Young's Internet Addiction Test (YIAT)

---

mood state, as opposed to promoting a positive value (such as the excitement of the game.) The deliberately endless nature of MMORPGs (sustained through "patches" to the game that alter the play universe in numerous ways) lends itself to continued game play. The gamer is also left with a sense of falling behind because the collective nature of the game dictates that others are advancing in the game. Increasing time played does not necessarily bring the end of a game. Sleep is lost, not only because of such extended play but also because the global nature of the game permits a user to play with opponents or collaborators anywhere in the world.

Griffiths (1996) offered six components for a behavior to be defined as addictive: salience (the behavior dominates thought, feelings, and behavior); mood modification (experiencing an arousing "buzz" or a paradoxically tranquilizing feeling of escape or numbing); tolerance; withdrawal; conflict (between addicts and those around them); and relapse. James displays many of these features. Griffiths further posited that addiction arises from a combination of biological predisposition, social environment, and psychological constitution.

TABLE 6–3. Suggested interview questions

Exploratory questions

What kinds of things do you do on your smartphone, tablet, laptop, or computer?

Do you have a game console, such as PlayStation, Nintendo, or Xbox?

Do you play massively multiplayer online role-playing games, such as *Final Fantasy*, *World of Warcraft*, or *Minecraft*?

Preoccupation

Do you find yourself thinking about gaming or anticipate the next time you will play?

Withdrawal symptoms

What do you experience when you cannot play?

Do you get restless, irritable, sad, or anxious if you are kept from playing or when you attempt to cut down or stop gaming?

Tolerance

Do you find that you need to play longer, or wish for more powerful equipment, for the same sense of excitement or relief?

Attempts to control participation

Have you ever tried to cut down how much or how often you play?

Loss of interests

What are some of the things you used to do for fun that you don't seem to have time or interest for any more?

Continued excessive use despite consequences

In what ways has online gaming cost you? Do you continue to play even though you are aware of these consequences?

Deception of others regarding gaming

How often do you hide from others or lie about the amount of time you are gaming?

Playing to escape or relieve a negative mood

Why do you play? Do you play to relieve feelings such as guilt, sadness, or anxiety?

Do you play to escape from personal problems?

Jeopardy or loss

Do you feel you have jeopardized or lost significant relationships, a job, or educational or career opportunities because of gaming?

Exclusion

Do you gamble online? Does any of your online play involve gambling?

Does any of your online play involve sexual Internet sites?

Severity

Help me understand the impact on your relationships and life.

How many hours do you spend on gaming?

Do you put off sleep so you can play more?

Do you skip meals to play more?

Source. Some questions adapted from Young's Internet Addiction Test by Kimberly Young and from Petry et al. 2014.

Why do young people play at all? Demetrovics et al. (2011) attempted to answer this question with their 27-item Motives for Online Gaming Questionnaire (MOGQ). Using a combined method of exploratory and confirmatory factor analysis, they described seven motivational factors: social, escape, competition, coping, skill development, fantasy, and recreation. The MOGQ offers 27 statements, such as "I play online games because gaming helps me to forget about daily hassles." These statements are rated from 1 to 5 (with respect to five intensity levels ranging from almost never/never to almost always/always).

Treatment

A lack of consensus in definition and assessment instruments, as well as of randomization and blinding procedures in the designs of the clinical trials for treatment of Internet gaming disorder, has contributed to the absence of evidence-based treatments. Currently, most treatments are offered on a case-by-case basis and are similar to other addiction treatments. These range from online educational programs and support groups to inpatient rehabilitation units. Individual psychodynamic therapy, cognitive-behavioral therapy, family therapy, group therapy, and pharmacotherapy have also been used in the treatment for Internet gaming disorder.

A comprehensive understanding of the patient's motivations is necessary for a broad treatment approach. In James' mind, gaming makes him feel good: In his virtual world, he accomplishes missions, gaines prestige and recognition, and makes friends he can relate to. He is able to present himself in any way he wants to through his avatar— he can be a priest or a knight or a healer. The intricacies of the game cater to his competitive side and contribute to building a tolerance. Every subsequent "level" takes more time and effort, but he is rewarded with more abilities and power. The virtual world persists even when James is not playing, and he often feels as though he is "missing out" and "falling behind" when he is not online.

James' chronic struggle with low self-esteem and social anxiety may be both impediments to treatment and anchor points for treatment; these symptoms lend themselves to traditional treatments, such as cognitive-behavioral therapy and dynamic therapies. The seminal case report by Keepers (1990) suggested that abstinence (due to residential placement) combined with individual and family therapies was effective for one preadolescent.

Studies in the neurobiology of Internet gaming disorder and other Internet addictions are just emerging, but they are in line with, for example, studies of cue-induced cravings in substance dependence, including a 10-participant functional magnetic resonance imaging study (Ko et al. 2009). Another study (Zhou et al. 2011) showed low gray matter density in the left anterior cingulate cortex of Internet-addicted adolescents when compared with healthy control subjects, in addition to low gray matter density in the left posterior cingulate cortex, left insula, and left lingual gyrus. One small study (Kim et al. 2011) showed decreased striatal dopamine D_2 receptor availability. Finally, a magnetic resonance imaging study of brain activity (Han et al. 2010) comparing patients with Internet video game addiction and healthy control subjects showed higher brain activation in the left occipital cuneus, left dorsolateral prefrontal cortex, and left parahippocampal gyrus in response to game cues. After a 6-week period of bupropion sustained-release medication, cravings for Internet video game play, total game play time, and cue-induced brain activity in the dorsolateral prefrontal cortex decreased in the Internet video game addiction group.

Conclusion

Inclusion of Internet gaming disorder among disorders for further study in DSM-5 should spur further research into the assessment and treatment of this debilitating behavioral addiction. Gambling disorder may be the first—but perhaps not the last—non-substance behavioral disorder to be recognized and documented.

Key Points

- Internet use should be queried in all psychiatric evaluations of children, adolescents, and young adults, particularly urban males.

- Internet gaming is not limited to nighttime computer sessions but is ubiquitously accessible, for example, on smartphones.

- Functional impairment is best explored by questioning change in overall behavior but particularly by assessing those activities and relationships that have been negatively affected.

- Massively multiplayer online role-playing games are associated with significantly more impairment than other types of Internet gaming.

- Assessment tools consist of multiple instruments, including an international consensus document offering nine statements probing each proposed DSM-5 criterion in the 11 main languages of countries with the most abundant research.

References

Achab S, Nicolier M, Mauny F, et al: Massively multiplayer online role-playing games: comparing characteristics of addict vs non-addict online recruited gamers in a French adult population. BMC Psychiatry 11:144, 2011

American Medical Association Council on Science and Public Health: Emotional and Behavioral Effects of Video Games and Internet Overuse, Report 12-A-07, 1–10, 2007. Available at: http://www.ama-assn.org/ama/pub/about-ama/our-people/ama-councils/council-science-public-health/reports/2007-reports.page?

American Psychiatric Association: Diagnostic and Statistical Manual of Mental Disorders. 4th Edition, Washington, DC, American Psychiatric Association, 1994

American Psychiatric Association: Diagnostic and Statistical Manual of Mental Disorders. 5th Edition. Arlington, VA, American Psychiatric Association, 2013

Brookhaven National Laboratory: The first video game? William Higinbotham's video game. Available at: http://www.bnl.gov/about/history/firstvideo.php. Accessed February 4, 2014.

Demetrovics Z, Urbán R, Nagygyörgy K, et al: Why do you play? The development of the motives for online gaming questionnaire (MOGQ). Behav Res Methods 43(3):814–825, 2011 21487899

Entertainment Software Association: Essential facts about the computer and video game industry, 2013. Available at: http://www.theesa.com/facts/pdfs/esa_ef_2013.pdf. Accessed September 22, 2014.

Goldberg IK: Internet addictive disorder (IAD) diagnostic criteria, 1995. Available at: http://www.psycom.net/iadcriteria.html. Accessed March 31, 2014.

Griffiths M: Nicotine, tobacco and addiction. Nature 384(6604):18, 1996 8900263

Han DH, Hwang JW, Renshaw PF: Bupropion sustained release treatment decreases craving for video games and cue-induced brain activity in patients with Internet video game addiction. Exp Clin Psychopharmacol 18(4):297–304, 2010 20695685

Keepers GA: Pathological preoccupation with video games. J Am Acad Child Adolesc Psychiatry 29(1):49–50, 1990 2295578

Kim SH, Baik SH, Park CS, et al: Reduced striatal dopamine D2 receptors in people with Internet addiction. Neuroreport 22(8):407–411, 2011 21499141

Ko CH, Liu GC, Hsiao S, et al: Brain activities associated with gaming urge of online gaming addiction. J Psychiatr Res 43:739–747 2009 18996542

Petry NM, Rehbein F, Gentile DA, et al: An international consensus for assessing Internet gaming disorder using the new DSM-5 approach. Addiction 109(9)1399–1406, 2014 24456155

Smahel D, Blinka L, Ledabyl O: Playing MMORPGs: connections between addiction and identifying with a character. Cyberpsychol Behav 11:715–718, 2008 18954271

Tao R, Huang X, Wang J, et al: Proposed diagnostic criteria for internet addiction. Addiction 105(3):556–564, 2010 20403001

Zhou Y, Lin FC, Du YS, et al: Gray matter abnormalities in Internet addiction: a voxel-based morphometry study. Eur J Radiol 79(1):92–95, 2011 19926237

Questions

1. Which of the following statements about online gamers is FALSE?

   A. Nearly 40% of online gamers consider themselves addicted.
   B. High levels of online gaming are also associated with high levels of off-line social support.
   C. There is a positive correlation between online game addiction and conduct problems.
   D. While most online game players are male, females are well represented at greater than 10%.

   The correct answer is B.

   Online gamers who spend more time on massively multiplayer online role-playing games (MMORPGs) have low levels of off-line social support. They display high levels of anxiety and depression and rate themselves lower for life satisfaction. Achab et al. (2011) citing the study by Smahel (2008) of an international cohort of gamers, which included 15.4% females, noted that almost 40% frequently identified themselves as addicted. Online gaming addiction has been found to be positively correlated with conduct problems in several studies.

2. Which of the following geographic areas has the highest prevalence of Internet gaming disorder?

   A. Asia.
   B. Europe.
   C. North America.
   D. South America.

   The correct answer is A.

   China and South Korea appear to be overrepresented among online gamers, as well as among those with problematic use.

3. Which of the following demographic characteristics of adult players of MMORPGs is FALSE?

   A. More likely to be male.
   B. More likely to be single.
   C. More likely to live alone.
   D. More likely to be unemployed.

The correct answer is D.

The typical adult MMORPG player is a single young male, living alone. He tends to be educated and employed. In a French study, players were more than twice as likely to live in an urban versus a rural area. About one-third of video game players are under 18 years of age.

CHAPTER 7

Internet Addiction

The Case of Henry, the "Reluctant Hermit"

Sean X. Luo, M.D., Ph.D.
Timothy K. Brennan, M.D.
Justine Wittenauer, M.D.

CASES of Internet addiction (IA), also known as problematic Internet use, began to appear in the literature in the early 1990s. Since then, this clinical entity has attracted significant attention from both clinicians and the popular media. In DSM-5 (American Psychiatric Association 2013), Internet gaming disorder is listed as a condition warranting more clinical research and experience (Section III). However, behavioral addiction phenomena encompassing the pervasive experience of the Internet itself, and not just the effects of online gaming, are not listed. Nevertheless, both anecdotal and systematic examinations of this phenomena point to some common, and possibly classifiable, features across different cultures and symptom subtypes (Block 2008).

Internet use can be viewed as a multifaceted reinforcing agent. Commonly reinforcing elements of its usage include multiplayer games, Internet pornography and virtual sex, online gambling, online shopping, and online communities such as chat rooms and bulletin boards. These features may interact with other behaviorally reinforcing elements, some of which are further delineated in other chapters in this book, which are not directly part of the Internet but are made more accessible or engaged in through the Internet, such as social networking. The emergence of social networking and other Web 2.0 applications have enhanced the immediacy and responsiveness of the Internet experience, and excessive use of social networking Web sites and applications is of growing concern. Regardless of the behavioral phenomenology, the underlying functional impairment often has several common features: withdrawal from social and occupational activities, increasing use and time spent despite attempts to cut down, and financial and social consequences of use. Clinicians familiar with dealing with substance use disorders will find similar themes within IA.

While the prevalence of IA is difficult to estimate, broadly inclusive studies (Aboujaoude et al. 2006; Bakken et al. 2009; Park et al. 2008) across different cultures indicate that a large fraction (3.7%–13% in the United States, 1%–5.2% in Norway, 10.7% in South Korea) of the Internet user population express at least some symptoms of excessive Internet use, and about 1% of Internet users have symptoms significant enough to warrant a diagnosis. Because IA disorder is often complicated by elements of other behavioral addictive phenomena, shame and denial are common and complicate estimates of morbidity. Furthermore, systematic reviews point to common psychiatric comorbidities such as depression, anxiety, symptoms of attention-deficit/ hyperactivity disorder (ADHD), obsessive-compulsive disorder (OCD), and hostility/aggression (Ko et al. 2012; Park et al. 2008). A number of factors have been identified to be significantly associated with IA, including male gender, younger age, drinking behavior, family dissatisfaction, university education, and recent stressful events (Bakken et al. 2009; Lam et al. 2009). While currently there is no unifying set of criteria for identifying and consolidating this group of patients for large-scale clinical studies, recent progress has been significant in ameliorating this growing global public health problem.

Clinical Case

Chief Complaint

"I just want to get out of the house."

History of Present Illness

Henry is a 31-year-old single, white man, currently living alone in an apartment in the New York Metropolitan Area. He works as a technical consultant for a health care company. He presents to a psychiatric office for consultation regarding significant subjective distress. From further discussion, it is apparent that his mother's insistence for the past 3 weeks has compelled him to seek psychiatric treatment. He reports that he is a generally a nervous person, not deriving much enjoyment from interpersonal connection, and that he feels anxious in most social situations. His current job, which "fits my night owl lifestyle perfectly," consists of working on various computer projects as a programmer on a flexible, deadline-driven schedule. He talks to his immediate supervisor 2–3 times a week, often over the phone, and submits his code over e-mail. He has had a long-standing problem with using the Internet as a source of comfort and "escape" from his work, which he describes as "a bore." His problems are mostly twofold. First, he is heavily involved in several online communities devoted to open-source projects of various types. He collaborates with other programmers around the world in building a variety of software applications, many of which he admits are "a waste of time—I do it just to have some fun." He reports liking the fact that he gets quick responses on bulletin boards and can discuss ideas with other members with ease, not having to "think about computers like my boss does." However, he reports that he has been checking these boards excessively, often spending hours and getting into heated online fights over minute, arcane technical controversies and working on these projects to his complete exhaustion. He obsessively reads "both mainstream and hacker" blogs, spending hours at a time to stay updated on the latest developments in hardware and software so that "my beta today doesn't become legacy tomorrow." He reports that his best friends reside in this "geek culture" of this particular software system that they are developing and that "it's going to be bigger than iTunes…and free!" When he doesn't get a chance to check the bulletin boards and blogs for a few days, or fight with several team members, he reports "compulsions" to go back, and he feels a significant amount of unease that he cannot extract himself from "useless hours of work that gets me nothing." He tried deleting his account, only to open a new account a few days later. Aside from what he calls "addiction to the Internet," he also states that he has a "porn addiction."

The only time he gets away from the bulletin boards during Internet use is when he visits online pornography Web sites to stream pornographic videos. He masturbates during and after viewing pornographic videos, but as "almost an afterthought. I can just watch the videos on their own for hours and hours." Recently, he has started using Web sites that offer a paid subscription service that allows him to have virtual sex via Web cam. These kinds of services can be expensive for Henry, and as he spends more and more hours online, he notes that he has charged hundreds of dollars on his credit cards. Furthermore, he believes that this pattern of behavior generally decreases his sex drive and motivation to look for partnered sex. He endorses chronic feelings of low mood because "I have trouble functioning normally in society," as well as a strong desire for connection and a community, but he reports anxiety over his physical appearance ("Look at me, I'm a fat slob") and social skills ("I don't know how to talk to girls").

His main source of social interaction includes his mother, who calls him frequently, and his ex-girlfriend—his only past romantic partner—who works as a teacher and has been trying to "drag me out of the house" for many years. Three months ago, his girlfriend decided to break up with him, citing his inability to commit to a marriage and his lack of "affection" for her. Henry reports that he was devastated by the news and wanted to reconcile with her but did not know how to do it. Furthermore, his girlfriend used to call him frequently to go out to a restaurant or see a movie, and though he never enjoyed these activities and preferred to interact with his online community instead, he usually begrudgingly agreed. Since the breakup, his girlfriend has stopped calling him, and he has felt trapped in his apartment with no reason to leave. He gets most of his food by ordering it online and has gained at least 10 lb in the past 2 months.

His schedule consists of staying up all night and sleeping all day; as he states, "I live in Manhattan, but I'm on Tokyo time." Lately, he has started to feel that his focus and concentration toward work have started to deteriorate, though "it's never been great. I procrastinate a lot." While he denies overt suicidal thoughts and feelings, he has started to feel "hopeless" because "I'm my own prisoner." He is several weeks behind on an important project at work, and although he is making up excuses to his boss, he is afraid they might terminate his contract at his upcoming review. He feels chronically mistreated, that "the world is always after little guys like me," and that his ultimately unsuccessful romantic relationship cements his idea that "I will always be just a geek." He feels ambivalent about his Internet use, saying that although he can see why his mother and ex-girlfriend think that it is a problem, his inverted schedule presents difficulties to interact effectively with others. He feels that "this is just who I am, and I don't want to have to change who I am so I can get married." On the other hand, he says, "I just want to break this cycle and become a normal person."

A comprehensive review of other psychiatric symptoms was otherwise not revealing. He denies manic or psychotic symptoms or other OCD symptoms. He denies using illicit substances, although in the past month he has started drinking more than his usual one or two beers per week, now often consuming three to six beers at a time a few times weekly. His self-reported 16-item Quick Inventory of Depression Symptoms score at intake was 15, and his 21-item Beck Anxiety Inventory score was 21. His 10-item Yale-Brown Obsessive Compulsive Scale score was 8.

Past Psychiatric History

Henry has a long-standing history of feeling shy and awkward around others. He reports that in high school he felt that he had a small group of intimate friends with whom he felt comfortable talking about technology and related topics, but he was never able to fit into the larger community and that "I just hated everyone." During junior year of high school, his grades deteriorated, and his parents found him isolated and irritable. They consulted a school counselor, and he visited a developmental pediatrician for an evaluation for ADHD. He was prescribed immediate-release methylphenidate that was quickly titrated to 30 mg/day with some subjective improvement. At the time he felt a profound sense of anhedonia and reported not feeling energetic enough to do all of his schoolwork. The methylphenidate allowed him to "work through" this apathy. He continued the medication for a few years until he was accepted into college, at which point he decided to self-discontinue his medication.

Henry's pattern of Internet use greatly increased when he moved away to college. He spent most of his free time with a small group of friends who shared common interests, and although his mood in college was generally good, he described several episodes of depressed mood related to dating stressors and searching for his first job. In both situations, these feelings lasted for a few months, and his friends noticed. During the period of trying to find a job, he noticed that his time spent on the Internet significantly interfered with his job search effort, often distracting him from filling out the appropriate paperwork and making arrangements for interviews.

He also believes that his lack of sexual desire for his ex-girlfriend may have had something to do with his preference to look for sexual satisfaction over the Internet. He wonders if his "moodiness" is in some way related to his Internet use, but the cause-and-effect relationship is difficult to disambiguate. During these "episodes," he did not seek psychological services because he feared that they would put him on ADHD medications, which he no longer wished to take, especially as his schoolwork continued to be satisfactory. He also reported that he was able to recover from these episodes after a few months, gradually returning to his baseline mood and function.

Other than using marijuana a few times, which he reports were generally positive experiences, he has not used any other illicit substances. His history of alcohol use also followed a similar pattern of escalation and de-escalation during these episodic mood instabilities. Although he reports that he liked to drink alcohol when he was at home by himself, he noted an increase in tolerance; he voluntarily cut down. No withdrawal symptoms were experienced.

Social History

Henry has a younger brother and was born in the suburb of a medium-sized Midwestern city. His parents are still married and living in the same city. His father is an accountant for a small local firm, and his mother works part-time as an educational consultant. He reports that his childhood was uneventful and that his parents are "stodgy" and "boring." He describes his younger brother as much more gregarious and physically attractive. He was a star swimmer in high school and is currently going to law school. His brother has also had more success in relationships and is now engaged to be married. He is often both resentful and admiring of his brother for both "getting the better hand genetically" and being "just overall a better guy than I am." Although his brother tries to reach out to him, he doesn't feels motivated to reciprocate.

Henry received generally good grades in high school and attended a well-regarded public university in the Midwest, graduating with a bachelor's degree in computer science. He subsequently gained employment at a technology firm as an entry-level engineer. His job required him to relocate to New York City 3 years prior to his arrival at the psychiatric office. At the time of the move, Henry was excited for the new opportunities he would find in Manhattan, specifically "finding friends and meeting more people." Regarding his dating life, Henry met his ex-girlfriend in college, and she also relocated with him to Manhattan in order to attend graduate school. He thinks that his relationship with her and her move to New York helped him tremendously in maintaining a good attitude. After she broke up with him, he felt despondent and hopeless.

Mental Status Examination

The mental status examination of the patient reveals the following: The patient is appropriately groomed, casually dressed, slightly overweight, and appears at his stated age. His behavior is mild-mannered and polite; he appears a little shy but maintains good eye contact. His speech is fluent and of normal volume, speed, and prosody. He describes his mood as, "I'm not feeling great." His affect is not notably dysphoric; he makes jokes at times during the interview. The patient's thought process is mostly linear, although at times ruminating and meandering. There is no evidence of disorganization or tangentiality. His recurrent thoughts follow the theme of "life is pretty pointless" and "I don't want to be a hermit, but this is who I am." The patient denies any suicidal ideation and any past suicide attempts. His insight and judgment appear to be fair; his intelligence is above average, based on his language and his academic achievements.

Discussion

Henry's case illustrates some of the typical features of this clinical entity. In most clinical scenarios, comorbidity with other psychiatric disorders exists in a large number of patients, making both diagnosis and management more challenging. One of the first objectives of the comprehensive psychiatric evaluation, therefore, is to establish the diagnosis as well as the severity and degree of functional impairment and to prioritize treatment goals.

Diagnostic Considerations

The exact diagnosis of IA remains problematic because there is no official list of criteria, and DSM-5 has yet to include it either in the main text or the appendix. There is no universally accepted diagnostic instrument for IA. Systematic reviews of various diagnostic instruments found that previous studies used inconsistent criteria, and these studies had significant methodological limitations (Byun et al. 2009). Several questionnaires have been designed to both diagnose and assess the severity of IA. The most commonly used instrument is the 20-item Young's Internet Addiction Test (Young 2010), which has been tested and validated in the United Kingdom, Finland, the United States, and other countries. Other validated instruments include the Chen Internet Addiction Scale developed in Taiwan, the Questionnaire of Experiences Related to the Internet developed in Spain, and the Compulsive Internet Use Scale developed in the Netherlands (for a review, see Beard 2005). Each of the assessment instruments has its unique advantages and disadvantages. The Chen Internet Addiction Scale was developed to be most inclusive, assessing behaviors across a wide spectrum of individuals who are unsure if they are Internet addicted and those who believe they know someone who is pathologically using the Internet. The Problematic Internet Usage Scale has the advantage of having seven subscales, each measuring an independent psychosocial dimension, including depression, loneliness, shyness, and self-esteem. These instruments often have different theoretical foundations and do not attribute the same causal factors to the IA phenomenon. Criticism is directed at some of the questionnaires because they attempt to characterize symptoms that are not related to addiction or addiction-like phenomena. Some questionnaires are explicitly designed to be self-reports and are adaptable to broad Web-based screening studies; these studies might therefore suffer selection bias and are not necessarily the most suitable for clinical evaluation purposes. Finally, an individual may manifest addiction behavior with some Web sites or specific Web applications but not to the entire Internet experience per se.

Given the lack of a definitive and universally agreeable set of criteria, we can adapt the current existing DSM-5 criteria for substance use (other) and extend it to IA (Table 7–1). The advantage of this approach is that immediate parallels can be drawn with most of the symptoms relating to other substance use disorders, and the clinical techniques in management and assessment of substance use disorders can be easily modified to address IA-related problems. Importantly, DSM-5 criteria likely have good cross-cultural applicability and validity, which may make it easier to adapt treatment programs to individuals from different cultural backgrounds.

The main differential diagnosis of IA involves the complex question of whether this phenomenon occurs as a comorbidity of an existing psychiatric disorder or as a consequence of one and, therefore, should not be regarded as an independent condition or the focus of clinical attention. Several studies have attempted to examine the underlying causes of IA. One study suggests that some patients use the Internet as a form of low-risk social interaction for those who are extremely fearful of conventional social situations (Campbell et al. 2006); another study suggests emerging IA may be related to a pathological coping strategy for adult developmental transitions and crises (Ko et al. 2006). Whereas extensive evidence for psychiatric comorbidity is well documented, the precise temporal and longitudinal order of events is not well characterized.

In the case of Henry, it appears that his IA symptoms occurred early in his life, and they are not exclusively coincident with episodes of his mood disorder (major depressive disorder versus dysthymic disorder), anxiety disorder (social phobia, possible generalized anxiety disorder), substance use disorder (alcohol use disorder), or ADHD. He also has never fully met the criteria for OCD. His IA symptoms appear to wax and wane, and they often worsen during symptomatic episodes of his other psychiatric conditions. This pattern of intertwined symptoms, exacerbating each other in a complex network of causal loop (Figure 7–1) is common. This constellation of psychiatric symptoms likely drives several psychosocial dysfunctions in both his work and personal life, and the occurrence and worsening of the symptoms, in turn, lowers self-esteem and capacity for self-control. The diagnostic evaluation therefore requires clear and careful attention to evaluate each of the putative comorbidities separately. When did the depressive symptoms begin? How do the symptoms correlate in time and in patterns of thoughts and behaviors? Did previous treatments for particular symptoms or disorders improve IA behaviors? Is there a prominent family history of another psychiatric disorder that can inform this diagnosis? In this case, at least from the information gathered from the initial diagnostic interview, Henry's IA cannot be easily described as only occurring as a part of another psychiatric condition. It therefore requires separate, but parallel, treatment with other psychiatric comorbidities.

As part of the differential diagnosis, it is important to rule out bipolar disorder, in which excessive Internet use may occur within a manic or mixed episode and which manifests as either an increased goal-directed activity or excessively

---

TABLE 7–1.   Proposed adapted diagnostic criteria for other (or unknown) substance use disorder: problematic Internet use

---

A. A problematic pattern of use of the Internet and other related technologies leading to clinically significant impairment or distress, as manifested by at least two or the following, occurring with a 12-month period:

1. Internet usage is in larger amounts of time or intensity than was intended.

2. There is a persistent desire or unsuccessful efforts to cut down or control use of the Internet.

3. A great deal of time is spent in activities necessary to use or recover from use of the Internet.

4. Craving, or a strong desire or urge to use the Internet.

5. Recurrent use of the Internet resulting in a failure to fulfill major role obligations at work, school, or home.

6. Continued Internet use despite having persistent or recurrent social or interpersonal problems caused or exacerbated by the effects of its use.

7. Important social, occupational, or recreational activities are given up or reduced because of Internet use.

8. Recurrent Internet use in situations in which it is physically hazardous.

9. Internet use is continued despite knowledge of having a persistent or recurrent physical or psychological problem that is likely to have been caused or exacerbated by Internet use.

10. Tolerance, as defined by either of the following:
    a. A need for markedly increased amounts of Internet use to achieve desired effect.
    b. A markedly diminished effect with continued same amount of Internet use.

11. Withdrawal, as manifested by the following: Internet use is at times employed to avoid withdrawal symptoms.

Specify if:

In early remission: After full criteria for problematic Internet use disorder were previously met, none of the criteria for problematic Internet use disorder have been met for at least 3 months but for less than 12 months (with the exception that Criterion A4, "Craving, or a strong desire or urge to use the Internet," may be met).

In sustained remission: After full criteria for problematic Internet use were previously met, none of the criteria for problematic Internet use disorder have been met at any time during a period of 12 months or longer (with the exception that Criterion A4, "Craving, or a strong desire or urge to use the Internet," may be met).

Specify if:

In a controlled environment: This additional specifier is used if the individual is in an environment where access to the Internet is restricted

TABLE 7–1.	Proposed adapted diagnostic criteria for other (or unknown) substance use disorder: problematic Internet use *(continued)*

Specify current severity:

   Mild: Presence of 2–3 symptoms.

   Moderate: Presence of 4–5 symptoms.

   Severe: Presence of 6 or more symptoms.

Source.   Adapted from the *Diagnostic and Statistical Manual of Mental Disorders,* 5th Edition. Arlington, VA, American Psychiatric Association, 2013. Used with permission. Copyright © 2013 American Psychiatric Association.

impulsive behavior. An equally important consideration is whether excessive Internet use occurs exclusively in the presence of the effect of another substance, such as stimulants or cocaine. Neither of these scenarios appears be applicable in the case of Henry. An additional consideration involves whether the clinical umbrella of IA is more useful than further categorization of Internet use behaviors by their respective purposes (Figure 7–2). For example, Henry's excessive use of pornographic sites can be a manifestation of his sexual addiction, although it appears that his obsession with sexual activity is somewhat circumscribed to the use of the Internet as an outlet, and he exhibits no other forms of sexual obsessions or compulsions. In this case, the patient's most prominent problem appears to be an overarching problematic use of the Internet across several applications, as well as a lack of ability to self-withdraw from his excessive Internet use.

Finally, as with other substance and behavioral use disorders, IA should be considered within the context of a comprehensive evaluation of personality disorders. Henry displays several traits of avoidant personality disorder and obsessive-compulsive personality disorder during the initial diagnostic interview. However, as treatment progresses, further personality characteristics may become more prominent, and as episodic symptoms resolve, the focus of clinical attention may shift to addressing long-standing dysfunctional patterns in behavior and interpersonal relationships.

Social and Cultural Considerations

One of the seminal features of IA relates to the prosocial characteristics of the behavior itself. The relationship between contemporary "geek culture" and "hacker culture" communities and behavioral pathology is still poorly understood. The complex relationship between alienation and striving for belonging and assimilation undoubtedly plays a unique role in the pathogenesis of IA phenomena. In our patient, his poor social functioning in adolescence and feelings of ostracism prompted him to avoid real-life relationships, which likely exacerbated his symptoms.

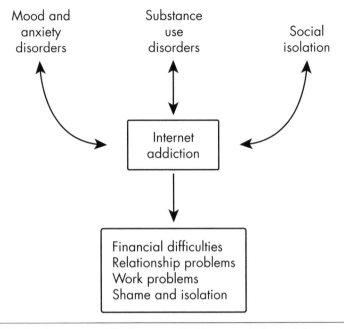

FIGURE 7–1. Internet addiction contributing psychological factors.
Internet addiction is commonly comorbid with mood and anxiety disorders, social isolation, and substance use disorders. The combination of these psychopathologies generates a variety of psychosocial problems that significantly impair normal functioning.

Different cultures have differing attitudes toward technology and Internet use. For instance, in a cross-cultural study comparing female students' attitudes toward Internet use, Chinese students reported more favorable attitudes toward computers and the Internet compared with British students (Li et al. 2001). Henry's family and immediate social surrounding may be less accepting of using the Internet as a legitimate means of interpersonal communication. This may cause additional shame and resentment that could potentially worsen disturbances in thoughts and behavior. Careful attention to the attitudes of the patient's families and communities toward Internet use is therefore an especially valuable part of the evaluation and can inform treatment and augment alliance. Whereas there is significant concern among parents and older individuals regarding problematic Internet use among children and young people, it is unclear whether these concerns are perhaps biased, because many parents grew up without any type of Internet or social networking. Whether these concerns dampen over time as a new generation of Internet-era parents comes of age remains to be seen.

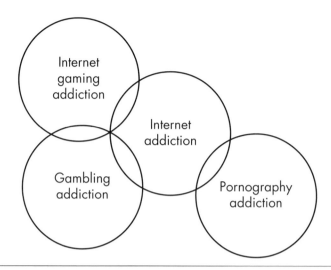

FIGURE 7–2. Internet addiction phenotype.

In clinical experience, Internet addiction is commonly overlapping and comorbid with a number of other behavioral addiction disorders such as pornography addiction (i.e., Internet pornography addiction), gambling addiction (i.e., addiction to online casinos and related behaviors), and Internet gaming addiction.

Treatment

Because of the lack of consistency and cross-cultural aspects of IA, interventional studies are often difficult to compare with each other. Nevertheless, the prevalence and potential degree of dysfunction have prompted a number of treatment studies. These studies evaluated a range treatment options, but they are often derived from distinct theoretical foundations. Currently, there is no consensus-based clinical guideline available for the treatment of IA, and there are no pharmacotherapy agents approved by the U.S. Food and Drug Administration for IA. Treatment is therefore primarily symptom-focused, with the goal of recovery being the improvement of the critical cognitive and psychosocial functioning that was significantly impaired by the behavioral disturbances. Some high-profile addiction treatment facilities have begun to enter the market for inpatient private-pay IA services.

Psychopharmacology

In order to identify pharmacological agents efficacious in modifying thoughts and behavior, the underlying circuit-level abnormalities should first be reviewed. Functional magnetic resonance imaging studies of IA subjects in China revealed a number of changes in these patients, including increased synchronization between the cerebellum, brainstem, limbic areas, and frontal cortex, indicating a potential role in the reward-processing pathways (Liu et al. 2010). Medications that potentially target reward and reinforcement may therefore have some effect on Internet use patterns. At the same time, because of the high degree of comorbidity, treating coexisting disorders may also improve the patient's IA symptoms.

Antidepressants

Antidepressant medications, particularly selective serotonin reuptake inhibitors, have a potential role in the treatment of IA, because the episodic comorbidity between IA and depression is high. Early case studies using escitalopram in the treatment of IA have resulted in anecdotal reports of improvement in mood and a reduction of craving for Internet use. In an open-label study (Dell'Osso et al. 2008) of 19 patients with 10 weeks at a uniform dose of 20 mg/day of escitalopram, 11 patients (64.7% of the sample, factoring in dropouts) had a significant decrease in weekly hours spent online and improvements in global functioning. At the end of the 10 weeks, participants were randomized to either continue escitalopram or receive a placebo. Clinical improvement remained in the second phase of the study, but no significant differences were observed between those who continued taking the drug and those who were switched to placebo. Long-term effects of antidepressants in patients with mild to moderate depression and IA have not been evaluated, and clinicians need to be especially vigilant in monitoring for activation and manic-switching side effects during antidepressant treatments, which can worsen IA behavior.

Opioid Receptor Antagonists

The possible overlap between IA, substance use disorders, pathological gambling, and sexual compulsions suggests that a common circuit-level abnormality may be involved. An especially attractive candidate circuit may be the prefrontal-limbic-striatal circuit that is prominently involved in the recognition and modulation of reward and reinforcement behaviors. Dopamine is the central neurotransmitter that has several putative roles in this circuit, from indicating reward itself to measuring error in estimated reward. Several agents have been developed to target the dopaminergic pathway in both the striatum and the cortex to treat substance use disorders. Opioid receptor antagonists inhibit dopamine release in the nucleus accumbens and ventral pallidum, they have been shown to be efficacious for opioid and alcohol use disorders, and they may have a potential role in the treatment of IA. The medical literature is currently limited to a single case report of successful treatment with naltrexone (150 mg/day) added to a stable dose of sertraline, which induced a 3-year remission (Bostwick and Bucci 2008).

Mood Stabilizers

Mood stabilizers may be efficacious in IA in targeting the potential overlap between symptoms in mania and IA. Some mood stabilizers, such as topiramate, may have a generalized antireinforcement effect, and they have been used in alcohol-dependent patients with varying clinical effect. Other mood stabilizers, such as lithium and valproate, may theoretically have some utility in treating pathological gambling. However, at present, the effectiveness of mood stabilizers in IA treatment has not been investigated in controlled studies.

Antipsychotics

Because atypical antipsychotics, similar to selective serotonin reuptake inhibitors, also target the serotonergic circuit, they have been investigated, especially as an augmenting agent in treating compulsive-impulsive spectrum psychopathologies, such as OCD. Several atypical antipsychotics have been shown to be effective in trichotillomania, skin picking, and borderline personality disorder. A single case study (Atmaca 2007) revealed that quetiapine (200 mg/day), gradually added to citalopram, improved IA symptoms in a 23-year-old patient. These improvements were maintained at a 4-month follow-up. The possible role of antipsychotics in the treatment of IA symptoms requires additional studies.

Psychostimulants and Other Medications

Because of a significant comorbidity between ADHD and IA, psychostimulants have been proposed as a possible treatment, especially for children and adolescents. A recent open-label trial of osmotic release oral-formulation (mean daily dose 30.5 mg) methylphenidate in 62 medication-naïve children with comorbid ADHD and Internet video game addiction reported a significant improvement in both ADHD symptoms and Internet use after 8 weeks of treatment (Han et al. 2009). Medications that indirectly act on ADHD symptoms, such as α_2 agonists (guanfacine, clonidine) may also have an effect on IA symptoms, although there is currently no controlled evidence supporting their use. Finally, emerging glutamatergic agents may have a role in targeting impulsive behaviors.

Psychotherapy

A number of studies and reviews for the psychosocial treatment of IA have been published (e.g., Huang et al. 2010; Winkler et al. 2013). For the most part, psychotherapy for these patients involves developing and maintaining skills important in self-limiting Internet use, as well as strategies for coping with cravings and social isolation.

Cognitive-Behavioral Therapy

At present, cognitive-behavioral therapy (CBT) is the mainstay of psychotherapy treatment for IA, and almost all existing trials include some component of CBT in their treatment program. CBT relies on recognition of maladaptive patterns and modification and reconstruction of distorted thoughts and behaviors. Skills often acquired as part of the CBT program include time management strategies, a more balanced view of the benefits and potential harms of the Internet, increased self-awareness and awareness of others and one's surroundings, identifying "triggers" of Internet "binge behavior," and increased capacity for managing emotions and cravings. In a trial of online counseling in 114 clients diagnosed with IA (Young 2007), most patients showed significant improvement by the eighth session, and symptomatic control was sustained at the 6-month follow-up.

Motivational Interviewing

Motivational Interviewing (MI) is a patient-centered and directive counseling approach for eliciting behavioral change. It assumes that the patient ultimately has the responsibility to change. The physician's role is to provide guidance and realistically assess the pros and cons of different choices; the physician engages the patient's intrinsic motivation for changing behavior. This approach has been demonstrated to be effective for a number of substance use disorders, and analogies drawn between illicit substance use and problematic Internet use can be made such that MI can be used effectively as a psychotherapy modality. Orzack et al. (2006) used a combination of CBT and MI in treating patients who engage in excessive Internet use and found that whereas the effect on total use time is not apparent, there is improvement in overall quality of life and symptoms of depression. As an example, in our case, we can try to help Henry consider different life goals and how they may be misaligned with his problematic Internet use. Whereas the Internet allows him to have a risk-free social life, his desires for relationships in real life and success in his employment can be used to self-motivate a potential change in behavioral patterns.

Psychodynamic Psychotherapy

Although there are no published controlled studies on the efficacy of psychodynamic psychotherapy in IA, this phenomenon can be conceptualized within the psychodynamic framework to design a customized therapeutic program for individual patients. In our case, Henry's main complaints about control, entrapment, and subsequent dysfunction can be explained and understood through recognition of a repeated pattern of behavior that may have an origin in his childhood, with his attachment response modeled specifically to patterns of his parents. The goal of this type of therapy is to engage the patient in understanding these difficult interpersonal patterns and to view IA as a manifestation of their own inability to deal with intimate relationships because of their earlier life experiences. Henry must consider possibilities to resolve these conflicts either internally or experientially through better communication with his family and friends. Psychodynamic approaches may be especially helpful in exploring his sexual feelings associated with using the Internet and his Internet use as a means of relieving tension and as a substitute for his lack of romantic partnership.

Integrative Approaches

Integrative psychotherapy attempts to use elements of different therapeutic approaches in a flexible, solution-focused way to help patients achieve their individual goals. Patients with substance use disorders often benefit from a flexible treatment program because treatment goals and directions change as treatment progresses. Often individual patients are not interested in changing at the outset, or he or she has a psychopathology such as depression that makes it too difficult to address the other problematic behavioral patterns. The initial approach may be pharmacologic, and as the patient's depressive symptoms begin to lift, he or she becomes more amenable to considering changing patterns of behavior that he or she often relies on for self-soothing. MI engages these patients and enhances this motivation and subsequently can improve the efficacy of CBT, which is most helpful when patients are fully committed to change and need a program to specifically adopt change in their lives and to monitor the progress that they have made. A randomized trial (Du et al. 2010) studied the effect of multimodal intervention in 56 adolescents with IA, comparing an eight-session group CBT intervention plus family sessions and psychoeducation workshops with a wait list control. Although Internet use decreased in both groups, symptomatic improvement was more pronounced in the treatment group.

Other Treatments

Group Therapy

Group therapy is commonly used in substance us disorders. Its effectiveness in treating IA has been mixed in controlled studies (Huang et al. 2010). The advantage of group therapy lies in the ability of the individual to acquire social skills in a real-world context and the possibility of improving and resolving shame, guilt, and isolation through sharing with others with similar experiences. There is no formal controlled study for 12-step facilitation treatment for IA, although these groups do exist in the community, often intermingling with groups for other behavioral addictions, such as sex addictions. In clinical practice, group therapy can often be an important and practical adjunct treatment modality for patients with IA symptoms.

Family Therapy

Family therapy and network therapy are likely an important aspect of treatment for IA. The approach is both informative and interventional. First, family members may be relieved to know that the symptoms that they recognized in their loved ones may be alleviated by becoming aware that IA is partially mediated by a causal loop that involves depression and anxiety, abnormalities that may be addressed through pharmacotherapy. Second, a powerful message of hope can be communicated: even persistent, dysfunctional patterns of behavior can be changed through commitment and treatment with psychotherapy.

Conclusion

Developing a standard of practice for the treatment of IA is still in its infancy. Because IA is not a currently accepted diagnosis in DSM-5, we do not yet know if IA is even a valid disease state. Current approaches rely mainly on anecdotal evidence and a preliminary understanding of sociobiological causal factors of this phenomenon. Existing literature and clinical experience suggest that in designing a treatment program for these patients, several elements are essential. First, treatment of psychiatric comorbidities such as anxiety and depression and other substance use disorders is an important element. Second, there is good evidence that a CBT program incorporating elements of restructuring distorted thinking and promoting active behavioral change can be effective. Third, involving family and other social support networks can be useful and effective.

Key Points

- IA can be conceptualized as a clinical entity that involves excessive Internet use that spans different domains and applications, that causes significant social and occupational dysfunction, and that produces symptoms common to other substance use disorders, such as craving and withdrawal.

- IA may be increasingly common and is a growing public health concern.

- Differential diagnosis of IA involves a careful assessment of potential comorbid psychiatric conditions.

- Treatment of IA should address both the symptom of excessive Internet use as well as the psychiatric comorbidities.

References

Aboujaoude E, Koran LM, Gamel N, et al: Potential markers for problematic Internet use: a telephone survey of 2,513 adults. CNS Spectr 11(10):750–755, 2006 17008818

American Psychiatric Association: Diagnostic and Statistical Manual of Mental Disorders, 5th Edition. Arlington, VA, American Psychiatric Association, 2013

Atmaca M: A case of problematic Internet use successfully treated with an SSRI-antipsychotic combination. Prog Neuropsychopharmacol Biol Psychiatry 31(4):961–962, 2007 17321659

Bakken IJ, Wenzel HG, Götestam KG, et al: Internet addiction among Norwegian adults: a stratified probability sample study. Scand J Psychol 50(2):121–127, 2009 18826420

Beard KW: Internet addiction: a review of current assessment techniques and potential assessment questions. Cyberpsychol Behav 8(1):7–14, 2005 15738688

Block JJ: Issues for DSM-V: Internet addiction. Am J Psychiatry 165(3):306–307, 2008 18316427

Bostwick JM, Bucci JA: Internet sex addiction treated with naltrexone. Mayo Clin Proc 83(2):226–230, 2008 18241634

Byun S, Ruffini C, Mills JE, et al: Internet addiction: metasynthesis of 1996-2006 quantitative research. Cyberpsychol Behav 12(2):203–207, 2009 19072075

Campbell AJ, Cumming SR, Hughes I: Internet use by the socially fearful: addiction or therapy? Cyberpsychol Behav 9(1):69–81, 2006 16497120

Dell'Osso B, Hadley S, Allen A, et al: Escitalopram in the treatment of impulsive-compulsive Internet usage disorder: an open-label trial followed by a double-blind discontinuation phase. J Clin Psychiatry 69(3):452–456, 2008 18312057

Du YS, Jiang W, Vance A: Longer term effect of randomized, controlled group cognitive behavioural therapy for Internet addiction in adolescent students in Shanghai. Aust N Z J Psychiatry 44(2):129–134, 2010 20113301

Han DH, Lee YS, Na C, et al: The effect of methylphenidate on Internet video game play in children with attention-deficit/hyperactivity disorder. Compr Psychiatry 50(3):251–256, 2009 19374970

Huang XQ, Li MC, Tao R: Treatment of Internet addiction. Curr Psychiatry Rep 12(5):462–470, 2010 20697848

Ko CH, Yen JY, Chen CC, et al: Tridimensional personality of adolescents with Internet addiction and substance use experience. Can J Psychiatry 51(14):887–894, 2006 17249631

Ko CH, Yen JY, Yen CF, et al: The association between Internet addiction and psychiatric disorder: a review of the literature. Eur Psychiatry 27(1):1–8, 2012 22153731

Lam LT, Peng ZW, Mai JC, Jing J: Factors associated with Internet addiction among adolescents. Cyberpsychol Behav 12(5):551–555, 2009 19619039

Li N, Kirkup G, Hodgson B: Cross-cultural comparison of women students' attitudes toward the Internet and usage: China and the United Kingdom. Cyberpsychol Behav 4(3):415–426, 2001 11710267

Liu J, Gao XP, Osunde I, et al: Increased regional homogeneity in Internet addiction disorder: a resting state functional magnetic resonance imaging study. Chin Med J (Engl) 123(14):1904–1908, 2010 20819576

Orzack MH, Voluse AC, Wolf D, et al: An ongoing study of group treatment for men involved in problematic Internet-enabled sexual behavior. Cyberpsychol Behav 9(3):348–360, 2006 16780403

Park SK, Kim JY, Cho CB: Prevalence of Internet addiction and correlations with family factors among South Korean adolescents. Adolescence 43(172):895–909, 2008 19149152

Winkler A, Dörsing B, Rief W, et al: Treatment of Internet addiction: a meta-analysis. Clin Psychol Rev 33(2):317–329, 2013 23354007

Young K: Internet addiction over the decade: a personal look back. World Psychiatry 9(2):91, 2010 20671891

Young KS: Cognitive behavior therapy with Internet addicts: treatment outcomes and implications. Cyberpsychol Behav 10(5):671–679, 2007 17927535

Questions

1.   Commonly comorbid psychiatric diagnosis for Internet addiction (IA) includes all of the following EXCEPT

   A. Major depressive disorder.
   B. Generalized anxiety disorder.
   C. Attention-deficit/hyperactivity disorder.
   D. Bipolar disorder.

   The correct answer is D.

   Although excessive Internet use can be a presenting symptom for a manic episode, IA is more commonly seen as comorbid with depression, anxiety disorders, and attention-deficit/hyperactivity disorder.

2.   All of the commonly used standardized instruments assess severity of IA. Which of the following also has subscales that measure other associated symptoms?

   A. Young's Internet Addiction Test.
   B. Compulsive Internet Use Scale.
   C. Problematic Internet Usage Scale.
   D. Chen Internet Addiction Scale.

   The correct answer is C.

   Although each of the assessment instruments has its unique advantages and disadvantages, the Problematic Internet Usage Scale has the advantage of having seven subscales, each measuring an independent psychosocial dimension, including depression, loneliness, shyness, and self-esteem.

3.   Which of the following medications is approved by the U.S. Food and Drug Administration for the treatment of IA symptoms either alone or as an augmentation?

    A. Escitalopram.
    B. Naltrexone.
    C. Topiramate.
    D. None of the above.

The correct answer is D.

Although there is anecdotal evidence that naltrexone and topiramate may have symptom-specific efficacy for excessive Internet use, there are no controlled studies for their efficacy and tolerability. Selective serotonin reuptake inhibitors are efficacious for the depression symptoms commonly comorbid in patients with IA, but there are no specific indications for the use of selective serotonin reuptake inhibitors in the treatment of IA.

CHAPTER 8

Texting and E-mail Problem Use

TAUHEED ZAMAN, M.D.
DANIEL LACHE, M.D.

THE surge in the accessibility, affordability, and convenience of computers and mobile phones over the past 20 years has altered the way in which we communicate with each other. Chats, tweets, texts, and e-mails have become part of life on an international scale. Electronic communication has connected families, strengthened friendships, and sparked marriages. Yet for some, the reliance on electronic devices may have unintended consequences.

In this chapter, we focus on the adverse consequences associated with texting and e-mail, because these have been identified as potential subtypes of problem Internet use in the research literature. Although problem Internet use is a term used interchangeably with Internet addiction in the literature, we will refer to problem Internet use rather than Internet addiction in accordance with recent changes in terminology for substance use and gambling disorders in DSM-5 (American Psychiatric Association 2013).

E-mail and texting share several features: they are electronic, private, and text-based modes of communication. They are asynchronous, allowing time for reflection before messages are submitted. Both can be done discretely in places where traditional modes of communication may be inappropriate. However, whereas text messages are generally limited to mobile phone devices, e-mail may be done through computer, laptop, or tablet. Another distinction is that text messaging is generally limited to 160 characters, whereas e-mail does not have a character limit (Table 8–1).

TABLE 8–1.   Characteristics of e-mail and texting

E-mail	Texting
Asynchronous	Asynchronous
Instantaneous	Instantaneous
Private and discrete	Private and discrete
Mobile phone or computer	Mobile phone only
Unlimited	Limit of 160 characters
Used more often for work	Used more often for personal relationships

Problematic e-mail and text use have been defined in different ways, making an assessment of prevalence difficult to determine. One study found that 34% of people reported checking their e-mail every 15 minutes or less (Renaud et al. 2006). In an AOL survey of 4,000 respondents, 15% self-reported as "e-mail addicted," many of whom reported checking e-mail first thing in the morning, at church, while driving, and in the middle of the night ("Think you might be addicted to email? You're not alone" 2007). With regard to texting, a Swedish study of young adults defined high text use as more than 20 messages per day and indicated that 4% belonged in this group (Thomée et al. 2011). Another survey of Taiwanese youth revealed that 16.7% met four or more adapted DSM-IV-TR (American Psychiatric Association 2000) criteria for dependence on mobile phones, which included text messaging behavior (Yen et al. 2008).

It appears that younger age raises the risk for problem phone use, which includes both e-mail and text messaging (Billieux et al. 2008). In addition, although women appear to text more frequently than men and exhibit more symptoms of problem use, men are at elevated risk for texting in dangerous situations, such as while driving.

Symptoms of problem e-mail and text use have been adapted from criteria established for substance use and gambling disorders (see Table 8–2). Among patients with problem phone use, one study reported that the most frequent symptom is withdrawal distress when one does not have access to the mobile phone (Yen et al. 2008). A substantial number of people in the Yen et al. study also reported experiencing "a marked increase in the frequency and duration of use to achieve satisfaction" as well as "using the mobile phone for longer or more frequently than intended." The most common functional impairment is relationship disturbance.

E-mail and text messaging may lead to other functional disturbances as well. High-intensity Internet users (who spend, on average, 50 minutes per day using e-mail) are more likely to report that their use affects sleep patterns, their ability to work, and their ability to meet people (Anderson 2001). Even for those who

---

TABLE 8–2.   Example criteria of problem e-mailing and texting behavior

---

E-mailing or texting more frequently or over a longer period than intended

Persistent desire or unsuccessful attempts to cut down or stop e-mailing or texting

Involvement in chronic behavior to e-mail and text or with efforts to access a device to do so

Cravings and urges to e-mail or text

Failure to fulfill obligations at work, home, or school because of e-mailing or texting behavior

Continuing to e-mail or text even when doing so causes social or interpersonal problems

Reduction or abandonment of social, occupational, or recreational activities because of e-mailing or texting

E-mailing or texting even when it is physically hazardous

Continuing to e-mail or text even when doing so may likely cause or exacerbate a physical or psychological problem

An increase in frequency or duration of e-mailing or texting to achieve satisfaction

Withdrawal symptoms (e.g., frustration, anxiety) or e-mailing or texting to avoid these feelings

---

Note.   Symptoms of problem e-mail and text use have been adapted from criteria established for substance use and gambling disorders.

do not spend excessive amounts of time with e-mail or text messages, there are times when use can be high risk. Hosking et al. (2009) found that drivers spend 400% less time looking at the road while text messaging, variability in lane positioning increases 50%, and missed lane changes increase 140%. There have been numerous reports of fatalities attributed to this phenomenon in the media, leading many states to ban the use of cell phones while driving.

Clinical Case 1: Joseph

Joseph is a 30-year-old, single man of Italian American background who presented to the clinic for follow-up after an inpatient hospital admission. He was admitted for 1 week for management of acute anxiety, suicidal ideation, and opiate dependence, following an altercation with his mother that required police intervention. At the time that Joseph arrived at the clinic he was sober for approximately 1 month, was taking citalopram and clonidine as prescribed at discharge, and voiced a desire for both ongoing medication management and psychotherapy. He endorsed symptoms of persistent, daily anxiety in a range of situations and identified this as a key trigger for his relapses into substance use in the past. He set goals of maintaining his sobriety and discussing a history of childhood sexual abuse, examining how this may have contributed to his anxiety and intermittent substance use throughout life, along with attendant family conflicts and legal difficulties. Joseph was diagnosed with generalized anxiety disorder and opiate use disorder in recent remission (action stage of change). He agreed on a schedule of regular, weekly visits for combined treatment.

During his initial visits, Joseph frequently removes his cell phone from his pocket as soon as he sits down across from the clinician. He answers all questions appropriately and makes intermittent eye contact, but he frequently returns to texting or sending e-mails throughout the sessions. Although distracted, Joseph appears genuinely invested in continuing treatment and openly discusses a number of issues including his history of trauma and addiction. When the clinician notes that Joseph seems at times to be distracted by his cell phone, he responds that he is texting friends ("we text more than we talk") or his girlfriend ("she gets anxious, and we just check in when I'm away"). The clinician inquires about other relationships in his life and learns that Joseph frequently relies on text messaging to communicate with friends and family, particularly family members with whom he has a history of conflict or who are aware of his early trauma. He prefers this to phone conversations or face-to-face encounters, which he acknowledges heighten his anxiety. He notes that since recently attaining sobriety, he feels more anxious in social situations and frequently picks up his cell phone to relieve this anxiety.

Over time, Joseph gains insight into the ways his trauma contributed to disturbed early attachments and later anxiety in social situations and relationships. He acknowledges the ways he uses the distraction of the cell phone to avoid direct interactions or intimate connection to others and to communicate asynchronously with friends and family in a way that enhances his sense of control. He feels this need for control and safety is a lifelong constant; he previously used substances as a means of feeling secure. The clinician notes that Joseph appears to manage his affect during sessions in the same manner, and Joseph agrees that the intimacy of psychotherapy sometimes feels like a trigger with respect to his history of trauma. These psychodynamic insights enhance Joseph's treatment by deepening the therapeutic relationship and strengthening his participation in motivational interviewing related to opiate use and maintaining sobriety. The combination of therapy and medication titration also leads to greatly reduced levels of anxiety. His cell phone use soon becomes a less frequent barrier during appointments and in his interactions with others. Apart from the emotion relief he experiences, his functionality improves to the point that he is able to attain employment without debilitating anxiety and to repair his relationship with his mother.

Clinical Case 2: Jane

Jane is a 23-year-old, single, African American woman with no prior psychiatric history who presented to the outpatient psychiatry practice complaining of anxiety interfering with her ability to accomplish tasks. Several months prior to her presentation, she experienced a breakup with a boyfriend. Around this time, she began to experience more anxious worry. She noted a recurring, intrusive thought that an intruder might enter her house and attack her, which led her to check the locks on her door with increased frequency. It started with checking a handful of times per day but has progressed to every half hour. Eventually, she started to wake up from sleep in order to check the locks. She reported being very distressed by this thought and recognized it as abnormal. However, each time the thought of an intruder occurred to her, the only thing that she could do to relieve the worry was to check the locks.

For 1 month prior to her presentation, Jane noticed that the anxiety began affecting her ability to perform her job. She noticed a recurring worry that she had missed someone's e-mail. She felt that this would lead to her missing something extremely important, so she checked her e-mail frequently. This checking was extremely time-consuming, because she needed to scroll down carefully through every message in her in-box until she ensured that each e-mail had been read previously. This typically consisted of hundreds of messages. After she finished this task, she would often start over again. Out of an 8-hour workday, Jane estimated that more than half of her time was spent going through her in-box. As a result, she neglected her other job duties and was on the verge of being fired.

At her initial visit, Jane is diagnosed with obsessive-compulsive disorder (OCD). Fluoxetine is prescribed, and Jane is referred to a therapist who specializes in exposure-response prevention (Foa and Goldstein 1978). In addition, Jane considers taking a temporary leave of absence from her employment. However, with her awareness of the cause of her impairment and the potential for treatment, she decides to let her employer know about her condition. Jane hopes that she will be allowed to continue to work at a reduced capacity. After receiving a letter from her physician, the employer agrees to allow her to continue at her job with a temporary reduction in workload.

During the first psychotherapy visit, Jane is given psychoeducation about OCD and taught how to keep a record of her symptoms. Triggers that lead to compulsive behaviors are identified. At the second visit, a hierarchy of distressing situations that were triggers for anxiety (e.g., using a computer at work that cannot receive e-mail) is created. These situations are gradually and systematically confronted between sessions, beginning with ones that are mildly distressing and progressing to those that are more distressing. In later visits, Jane is encouraged to repeatedly imagine and describe some of her worst fears. She also works on ritual prevention, which consists of experiencing distressing thoughts, which normally are relieved by ritualistic checking, and purposefully prevents herself from checking behavior. Throughout the treatment, her anxiety, thoughts, and behaviors are recorded and monitored. At first, Jane's confrontation of thoughts and situations that she was managing through compulsive behavior is extremely stressful. However, by the end of 12 weeks, she reports a significant improvement in anxiety, sleep, and functioning. She no longer feels impaired by compulsive behavior and is able to again accomplish all of her tasks at work.

Clinical Case 3: Terry

Terry is a 27-year-old, single, white man with a history of attention-deficit/hyperactivity disorder (ADHD) who was referred by his psychotherapist to the outpatient psychiatry practice for problems with inattention and impulsivity. He noted that these have been problems for him since early childhood, when it was extremely difficult for him to pay attention in class. He also endorsed an inability to sit still. Terry had difficulty waiting his turn and would often call out rather than raise his hand. This led to frequent trips to the principal's office. As he got older, Terry was placed in classes with lower-achieving students. Fights with his peers led to several suspensions from school. During his adolescence, Terry went to a child psychiatrist and was prescribed amphetamines. However, this led to a marked decrease in appetite, and he discontinued this medication after 1 week. He did not have subsequent experiences with psychiatrists or therapists.

Terry graduated from high school and was accepted into a community college. However, he lost interest in college after one semester and left. Since leaving college, Terry has had only intermittent employment. He has been fired numerous times for being late for or absent from work. He also noted that "forgetfulness" has impaired his ability to perform complex tasks in the workplace.

At the time of intake, Terry reports continued struggles with impulsivity and impatience, which have caused both legal and relationship issues. He has received numerous speeding tickets and endorses difficulty waiting his turn when on lines. He notes that his "hot temper" has led to both physical and verbal aggression with friends. After these episodes, Terry regrets his lack of control. He worries that he has burned all of his bridges and feels a painful sense of loneliness as a result.

In the office, Terry has marked difficulty giving a thorough history. He frequently takes out his phone and texts an unknown recipient. Terry struggles to answer open-ended questions from the psychiatrist, while at the same time engaging in a separate, text-based conversation. He is asked to place his phone aside so that the evaluation can be completed, and this leads him to begin to answer questions appropriately. However, after the phone vibrates, Terry picks it up again and checks the incoming text message.

After intake is complete, the psychiatrist collects collateral information prior to starting treatment. He first calls Terry's parents, who confirm the childhood diagnosis of ADHD and provide some additional details. They are extremely concerned that given Terry's history of impulsivity, he might wind up in jail for assault or in some sort of traffic fatality. Next, the psychiatrist reviews his psychotherapy notes, observing that "It was difficult to get patient's attention in session. He looked at his phone and sent texts several times a minute."

Terry begins a low dose of methylphenidate. At his next visit, he reports feeling somewhat more calm and focused. He has not acquired speeding tickets since the prior visit. Although he continued to feel irritable at times, there are no incidents of physical violence. Furthermore, he denies having side effects, including appetite suppression.

Terry's psychotherapist notes that he appears to be more engaged in session. However, Terry continues to be extremely distracted in session by his cell phone. The therapist points out that Terry cannot accomplish goals in therapy if he continues to be distracted by his phone. Terry agrees with this but reports that it is very hard for him to avoid checking his phone whenever it vibrates. He simply wants so much to know what the text message contains that he cannot delay reading it. Eventually, the therapist negotiates with Terry that the phone be kept off for most of the session. They will take a short break halfway through the hour, at which point the phone can be turned on briefly. Terry agrees. The rest of the sessions focus on supportive problem solving targeted to Terry's relationship, occupational, and legal issues, and coping strategies are developed for Terry to manage distress constructively. In addition, Terry is coached on cognitive and behavioral techniques for ADHD. Over the course of treatment, Terry is able to avoid legal difficulties. His improved focus as a result of medication and therapy allows him to stay at a new place of employment for an extended period of time. Eventually, he gains the ability to manage the inevitable frustrations in his relationships without damaging the relationships.

Management

Psychotherapy

Although no scientific studies to date have supported a mode of psychotherapy for treatment of problematic texting or e-mail use, literature suggests that screening for and addressing associated problems may prove useful. In particular, studies indicate that problem use of mobile phones (though not texting in particular) is associated with the personality trait of low self-esteem, although extraversion is associated with more intense use (Pedrero Pérez et al. 2012). Both text messaging and e-mail use may prove viable areas of therapeutic focus through the appropriate modality (psychodynamic therapy, cognitive-behavioral therapy, etc.). Studies have suggested that cognitive-behavioral therapy may have efficacy in treating problematic Internet use (Young 2007), although the degree to which this might apply to problematic text messaging and e-mail use remains unclear.

Other studies have suggested that cognitive limitations, emotional reactivity, depressive symptoms, peer influence, and trauma or negative life events may be associated with problematic mobile phone use (Billieux et al. 2008). Thus, screening for these issues (not to mention Axis I pathology) and tailoring psychotherapy appropriately may prove useful. In cases where emotional reactivity and trauma-related experiences appear pertinent, dialectical behavior therapy or other modes targeting these issues may prove useful. If, as in the cases presented, the patient has from an associated diagnosis (posttraumatic stress disorder, ADHD, OCD, etc.), management of these symptoms may relieve problematic texting or e-mail use.

Psychodynamically, problematic text messaging use in young people may stem from a desire to feel in better control of interactions and relationships with others (Madell and Muncer 2007). Texting and e-mail both allow individuals to communicate synchronously (i.e., in real time) or asynchronously (with whatever pauses in conversation are desired). The ability to communicate asynchronously in particular may give participants the sense of better control over interpersonal interactions, compared with face-to-face or telephone conversations. If this usage becomes pathological, patients may benefit from group therapy or other modes focused on enhancing social skills and comfort with interpersonal interactions outside of the texting and e-mail mediums.

Psychopharmacology

To our knowledge, no medications to date have been studied for the treatment of texting and e-mail problem use.

Psychoeducation

Patients, and families in the case of younger individuals, may benefit from education about the associations of problem use of texting and e-mail with the cognitive and emotional problems noted in the section "Psychotherapy." Additionally, studies have supported the association between problematic mobile phone use and the increased risk of traffic accidents (McCartt et al. 2006; Vivoda et al. 2008). Both patients and families may benefit from preventative counseling surrounding the risks associated with texting and e-mail use while driving, a risk that may be heightened in those who display problematic use in other spheres of their lives. Researchers have also noted a parallel increase in pedestrian injuries among mobile phone users (Nasar and Troyer 2013), and this may warrant attention. Education surrounding the developmental effects of cell phone use (as discussed in the section "Texting and E-mail Problem Use and Development") may also prove useful.

Texting and E-mail Problem Use and Development

Early studies indicate that problematic Internet use may be associated with characteristics of early parent-child bonding, mediated by the ways in which children learn to relate to others (Kalaitzaki and Birtchnell 2014). Additionally, early studies indicate that mobile phone use may affect cognition in adolescents (Abramson et al. 2009). In particular, adolescent mobile phone use may be associated with faster but more inaccurate responses to cognitive tasks.

Conclusion

The cases of Joseph, Jane, and Terry demonstrate the range of disorders that may be associated with problematic use of text messaging or e-mail. Other disorders may, in fact, bring the issue to clinical attention. It remains likely that problematic use of these technologies remains subclinical, largely undetected, and, therefore, unaddressed in a large number of individuals. This may explain the paucity of research in the field and the lack of clear, evidence-based criteria for diagnosis.

Nonetheless, because problematic texting and e-mail use can impede normal functioning or indicate underlying dysfunction in relating to others, patients struggling with this issue should receive appropriate management. In some cases, medication and psychotherapy for the associated depressive, anxiety, or other disorder may provide relief. Cognitive-behavioral therapy or psychodynamic work may also prove useful. Clinicians should educate young patients and their families about the cognitive effects of intensive use and the risk of accidents and injury associated with inappropriate use in some settings.

Some have theorized that problematic texting and e-mail use may stem from not just a desire for increased control over asynchronous interactions but also from a desire to escape from one's reality to live in an artificial, even if transient, safe environment (Collins 2014). In each case, an understanding of the social and cultural context in which problematic use occurs remains key to effective identification and treatment.

Key Points

- Problematic use of texting and e-mail has been defined in a number of ways. There is a relative lack of research on the topic and no formal diagnostic criteria in DSM-IV-TR or DSM-5.

- Problematic use of texting and e-mail may be associated with depressive, anxiety, or other disorders, which may warrant careful screening and management.

- Psychotherapy focused on addressing associated disorders and examining any interpersonal difficulties that underlie asynchronous communication may prove helpful.

- Patients, particularly adolescents, and their families should be advised regarding the impact on safety of texting and e-mail problem use.

References

Abramson MJ, Benke GP, Dimitriadis C, et al: Mobile telephone use is associated with changes in cognitive function in young adolescents. Bioelectromagnetics 30(8):678–686, 2009 19644978

American Psychiatric Association: Diagnostic and Statistical Manual of Mental Disorders, 4th Edition, Text Revision. Washington, DC, American Psychiatric Association, 2000

American Psychiatric Association: Diagnostic and Statistical Manual of Mental Disorders, 5th Edition. Arlington, VA, American Psychiatric Association, 2013

Anderson KJ: Internet use among college students: an exploratory study. J Am Coll Health 50(1):21–26, 2001 11534747

Billieux J, Van der Linden M, Rochat L: The role of impulsivity in actual and problematic use of the mobile phone. Appl Cogn Psychol 22(9):1195–1210, 2008

Collins M: Priory treats text addicts. Daily Mail Online. Available at: http://www.dailymail.co.uk/news/article-198547/Priory-treats-text-addicts.html. Accessed January 25, 2014.

Foa EB, Goldstein A: Continuous exposure and complete response prevention in the treatment of obsessive-compulsive neurosis. Behav Ther 9(5):821–829, 1978

Hosking SG, Young KL, Regan MA: The effects of text messaging on young drivers. Hum Factors 51(4):582–592, 2009 19899366

Kalaitzaki AE, Birtchnell J: The impact of early parenting bonding on young adults' Internet addiction, through the mediation effects of negative relating to others and sadness. Addict Behav 39(3):733–736, 2014 24368006

Madell DE, Muncer SJ: Control over social interactions: an important reason for young people's use of the Internet and mobile phones for communication? Cyberpsychol Behav 10(1):137–140, 2007 17305461

McCartt AT, Hellinga LA, Bratiman KA: Cell phones and driving: review of research. Traffic Inj Prev 7(2):89–106, 2006 16854702

Nasar JL, Troyer D: Pedestrian injuries due to mobile phone use in public places. Accid Anal Prev 57:91–95, 2013 23644536

Pedrero Pérez EJ, Rodríguez Monje MT, Ruiz Sánchez De León JM: [Mobile phone abuse or addiction. A review of the literature] [in Spanish]. Adicciones 24(2):139–152, 2012 22648317

Renaud K, Ramsay J, Hair M: "You've got email!"... shall I deal with it now? Electronic mail from the recipient's perspective. Int J Hum Comput Interact 21(3):313–332, 2006

Think you might be addicted to email? You're not alone. News Release, Investor Relations, AOL, July 26, 2007. Available at: http://ir.aol.com/phoenix.zhtml?c=147895&p=irol-newsArticle_print&ID=1354021&highlight=. Accessed January 11, 2014.

Thomée S, Härenstam A, Hagberg M: Mobile phone use and stress, sleep disturbances, and symptoms of depression among young adults—a prospective cohort study. BMC Public Health 11:66, 2011 21281471

Vivoda JM, Eby DW, St Louis RM, Kostyniuk LP: Cellular phone use while driving at night. Traffic Inj Prev 9(1):37–41, 2008 18338293

Yen CF, Tang TC, Yen JY, et al: Symptoms of problematic cellular phone use, functional impairment and its association with depression among adolescents in Southern Taiwan. J Adolesc 32(4):863–873, 2008 19027941

Young KS: Cognitive behavior therapy with Internet addicts: treatment outcomes and implications. Cyberpsychol Behav 10(5):671–679, 2007 17927535

Questions

1. Which of the following statements is TRUE?

    A. Age is not a factor for problem texting behavior.

    B. Women are at highest risk for problem texting behavior.

    C. Women text more frequently, but men are at higher risk for texting in dangerous situations.

    D. Depression is a protective factor for problem texting behavior.

The correct answer is C.

According to published research, younger age increases the risk for problem phone use. Although women appear to text more frequently than men and exhibit more symptoms of problem use, men are at elevated risk for texting in dangerous situations, such as while driving (Billieux et al. 2008). Depressive symptoms have been linked to problem phone use.

2. Which of the following is NOT a symptom of problem e-mail or texting behavior?

    A. Impaired relationships.
    B. Preference of iPhones over Android.
    C. Use despite potential harm.
    D. Distress when ability to check e-mails and texts is removed.

The correct answer is B.

Much of the literature regarding problem phone use (including e-mail and texting) has used adapted DSM-IV-TR dependence criteria, which include impaired functioning, use despite potential harm, and withdrawal distress (Yen et al. 2008).

3. Which of the following is TRUE regarding management of psychiatric comorbidities in patients with problem e-mail/phone use?

    A. A combination of psychopharmacology and psychotherapy may be helpful.
    B. A focus on the problem behavior without addressing comorbidities is preferred.
    C. Problem e-mail/texting behavior places people at lower risk for other disorders.
    D. Inpatient management is preferred because of high risk of danger to self.

The correct answer is A.

We have found an integrated approach to be most helpful for improving outcomes. This is particularly true given the lack of established psychopharmacologic and psychotherapeutic options for problem e-mail and texting behavior.

4.   Which of the following statements about adolescents and problematic texting/e-mail use is TRUE?

A. May be associated with difficulties on certain cognitive tasks.
B. May be associated with driving-related injuries.
C. May be related to interpersonal difficulties or anxiety.
D. All of the above.

The correct answer is D.

According to recent research, problematic text messaging/e-mail may be associated with inaccuracies on cognitive tasks (Abramson et al. 2009) and increased injuries among drivers/pedestrians (McCartt et al. 2006; Vivoda et al. 2008). Problematic use may also stem from interpersonal difficulties, which can be avoided because of the asynchronous nature of this medium (Collins 2014).

5.   Which of the following may be associated with problematic texting/e-mail use?

A. Symptoms of psychosis.
B. Symptoms of schizoid personality disorder.
C. Symptoms of depression or anxiety.
D. Symptoms of mania.

The correct answer is C.

Studies show that patients may experience symptoms of depression (among them, low self-esteem) and anxiety and may benefit from screening/management around these issues (Billieux et al. 2008; Pedrero Pérez et al. 2012).

CHAPTER 9

Kleptomania

To Steal or Not to Steal—
That Is the Question

Erin Zerbo, M.D.
Emily Deringer, M.D.

THE term *kleptomania* derives from the Greek roots *kleptein* and *mania,* meaning "stealing insanity." It was first coined as "klopemanie" in 1816 by a Swiss psychologist named Andre Matthey, who described the condition as "the compelling impulse to steal a worthless or unneeded object" (Marazziti et al. 2003, p. 36). Juquelier and Vinchon (1914) noted that "the thieving tendency triumphs, it subjugates the will" (p. 50). Two French physicians, C. C. Marc and Jean-Étienne Esquirol, slightly altered this term to "kleptomanie" in 1838 and noted the sense of exhilaration and relief of tension that those afflicted experienced during the act of theft. They described several cases of socially and economically elite persons, including European royalty, and emphasized that such shoplifting of trivial items was "involuntary and irresistible" and disproportionately affected females (Grant 2006). There was subsequently much debate in the psychiatric community about the validity of the diagnosis, yet, even as early as the 1830s, Esquirol himself was participating in the legal defense of upper-class women who were accused of shoplifting (Goldman 1991).

In these early years, the debate about kleptomania took place entirely within the psychoanalytic community. There were various case reports and extensive theorizing. It was listed as a "supplementary term" in 1952 in DSM-I (American Psychiatric Association 1952) but then removed entirely from DSM-II (American Psychiatric Association 1968). It was reinstated in 1980 in DSM-III (American

Psychiatric Association 1980) under "Disorders of Impulse Control Not Elsewhere Classified" and remained in this category ("Impulse-Control Disorders Not Elsewhere Classified") through the publication of DSM-IV-TR (American Psychiatric Association 2000). In DSM-5 (American Psychiatric Association 2013), this category was expanded and renamed "Disruptive, Impulse-Control, and Conduct Disorders." Pathological gambling and trichotillomania were removed from the impulse-control disorders (ICDs) category, and oppositional defiant disorder, conduct disorder, and antisocial personality disorder were all relocated here (antisocial personality disorder is dual coded and remains in the "Personality Disorders" section as well). See Box 9–1 for the current DSM-5 criteria for kleptomania, which remain unchanged from DSM-IV-TR.

Box 9–1. Diagnostic Criteria for Kleptomania

A. Recurrent failure to resist impulses to steal objects that are not needed for personal use or for their monetary value.
B. Increasing sense of tension immediately before committing the theft.
C. Pleasure, gratification, or relief at the time of committing the theft.
D. The stealing is not committed to express anger or vengeance and is not in response to a delusion or a hallucination.
E. The stealing is not better explained by conduct disorder, a manic episode, or antisocial personality disorder.

Source.   Reprinted from the *Diagnostic and Statistical Manual of Mental Disorders,* 5th Edition. Arlington, VA, American Psychiatric Association, 2013. Used with permission. Copyright © 2013 American Psychiatric Association.

As demonstrated in the case presentation, kleptomania is often seen with psychiatric comorbidities, and its varied manifestations may account for the reluctance of the psychiatric community to categorize it as a separate disorder in its own right. Yet, as we will see, there are definitive signs and symptoms that clearly distinguish kleptomania from other types of theft and other brands of compulsive behavior.

See Video 4 for a dramatization of the clinical encounter that follows. Note how the therapist remains neutral yet persistent in her attempts to help the patient open up about her shoplifting. Given the highly secretive nature of the disorder, patients are often reluctant to talk about the behavior at all, and clinicians should consider asking about it routinely during initial evaluations to indicate that they are familiar with it.

 Video Illustration 4: Kleptomania: getting the history (5:57)

Clinical Case

Sherry is a 35-year-old white woman with a history of recurrent major depressive disorder, generalized anxiety disorder, and a history of bulimia nervosa in her 20s (now mostly resolved); she has no significant past medical history aside from a diagnosis of irritable bowel syndrome. Sherry has been in outpatient psychiatric treatment several times since her early 20s, usually for a period of several months or at most 1 year. She has been prescribed antidepressants (both selective serotonin reuptake inhibitors [SSRIs] and serotonin-norepinephrine reuptake inhibitors) for her depressive and anxiety symptoms, as well as when her bulimia was more symptomatic. She has a history of cutting behavior in her teen years before she ever saw a psychiatrist but no self-injurious behavior in the past 15 years and no history of suicide attempts, nor has she ever been psychiatrically hospitalized. She has no formal history of a substance use disorder (SUD). Sherry has several extended family members with anxiety or depression and alcohol use disorders.

Sherry now presents to the outpatient mental health clinic at the urging of her husband, who has become increasingly distressed by her behavior. She has been arrested three times in the past year for shoplifting; each case has been dropped after they have spent considerable money on legal representation. Her husband was initially concerned and sympathetic, but he has now become angry with her, and her most recent arrest is causing significant discord in their marriage. She gave a rather superficial explanation after she was first arrested, telling him that she wasn't quite sure what had gotten into her and that it would not happen again; but now, two arrests later, he has tired of her repeated promises, and he is both annoyed and dismayed by the lack of any depth in her explanation. He has noticed that she has appeared dysphoric and more apathetic this year, but he is no longer sympathetic. He has threatened to separate from her if she doesn't seek psychiatric help immediately.

On the initial interview at the clinic, Sherry presents as a well-groomed, stylish woman wearing light makeup and delicate jewelry, with her hair pulled back into a neat braid. She is polite, although somewhat guarded and superficial, drawing her arms across her chest and answering the initial evaluation questions with only brief replies. She describes her situation without demonstrating much affect and notes that her primary reason for attending treatment is to appease her husband. She denies any current depressive or anxiety symptoms and replies curtly that her bulimia is "not a problem right now." She asks for a letter at the end of the evaluation so that she can prove to her husband that she attended the session.

Sherry dutifully returns for her second session, but she remains just as guarded as during the intake session. After asking several routine questions, the therapist begins to address her apparent indifference and to wonder aloud what might be behind it. The therapist asks her to speak a little bit more about her teenage years and her first interactions with a psychiatrist in her 20s, and her demeanor gradually begins to soften. She becomes tearful and describes depressive symptoms dating back to her teenage years and periods when her loneliness was compounded by paralyzing anxiety. She notes that medications have been helpful at various times, but she never felt especially connected to a psychiatrist or therapist, and "I never felt I really got anywhere with it," so she would discontinue treatment once she felt better. Often her primary care doctor would prescribe an antidepressant for her for a period of time afterward, and then she would discontinue it altogether.

Although it takes some time, the therapist is gradually able to approach the subject of her shoplifting. She becomes hesitant and soft-spoken and initially attempts to provide the same superficial explanations that she offered to her husband. Yet, after some time, she finally takes a deep breath and looks down sheepishly.

"You know, the truth is that I don't really understand it myself. Lately, it's gotten to the point that when I'm driving to the grocery store, it's practically all I can think about. It's like this exciting thing that is just mine… I'll just slip a few small items into my purse while I'm shopping, and no one will be the wiser. I get this big rush right before I do it, and sometimes I get careless or it's almost like I want to get caught—like not worrying about a security guard I just saw in the next aisle. And afterward, after I get through the check-out line and get out those front doors and I know that I got away with it—I feel really great for a little bit, like on top of the world. But pretty soon it all comes crashing down again, and I just feel guilt and remorse, asking myself why someone like me would be doing something so ridiculous. It's always silly stuff that I take, little things like tweezers or lip balm, but I can't even bear to look at them once I get home, and I just shove them in the back of the closet. Then I start to worry that my husband, Dan, will find them, this box of little random items tucked away in the closet, so I put them in a plastic bag and throw it all away, and I swear to myself that I won't do it again. I've made that promise to myself too many times to count. And the frustrating part is that I meant it every time."

Sherry goes on to describe that she first stole during her teen years, during a "dark period" in which she felt depressed and was cutting herself for relief. She did it on a whim her first time, and she was surprised how much it boosted her spirits. She shoplifted on and off during her teen years but then curbed the behavior in her 20s, although she did notice that it tended to come back again during periods when she felt more depressed. She felt she "had it under control" by the time she got married at 29, and she was proud that she had entirely stopped shoplifting.

"But then somehow it came back again these past few years…Dan has to travel a lot for his job, and I've just felt really lonely sometimes. I know my depression has been creeping back, but I didn't want to address it, I just wanted it to go away…and right on schedule, back came the shoplifting. It caught me by surprise. But I told myself it was so harmless and minor, no one would have to know. I didn't even feel much guilt or shame in the beginning. And it always seemed to make me feel better. But this year, it's just gotten entirely out of control, and I've been doing it in riskier situations, almost to increase the thrill or something— and now I've gotten arrested three times! It's just mortifying; I could have died when they walked me through the store to that back room and told me they were actually pressing charges. But somehow it still didn't stop me. That's the part that's so weird. How could I keep doing this even after that?"

Sherry notes that she never discussed this with prior therapists because of concern that she would "get in trouble." She was also worried that "it just seemed so weird, like I was a criminal or something, but it doesn't feel that way at all when I'm doing it." No psychiatrist or therapist had ever asked her about it, so she had never brought it up. Upon further discussion, it also becomes clear that Sherry has also been increasing her alcohol consumption over the past several years. She had periods of heavy drinking before (especially when more depressed), but lately, she has been drinking at least several glasses of wine most nights of the week. This had never been addressed during prior psychiatric treatment.

Discussion

Sherry probably represents the most "typical" case of kleptomania that we find in the literature, but this is a minimal literature, largely based on case reports and small studies, and there is no certainty about the "typical" patient with kleptomania. This is due to its hidden nature: it is a secretive disorder, often beginning in adolescence or early adulthood but not coming to clinical attention until the mid to late 30s, or perhaps even later for men (age 50). Many patients present for treatment because of legal coercion after being arrested for shoplifting, and the diagnosis is often missed in routine psychiatric evaluations. Individuals with kleptomania are often ashamed about their behavior, and the stolen items are usually hidden or discarded. Patients with kleptomania do not discuss it, even if they are already in psychiatric treatment, and clinicians do not usually inquire about it. One study found that only 42% of married individuals with kleptomania had even told their spouses about the behavior (Grant 2006).

Epidemiology

It is hard to know just exactly how many people have kleptomania, given its secretive nature. Although there has never been a national epidemiologic study conducted, the commonly quoted prevalence is 0.6% in the general population. However, this figure was extrapolated from combining data from two separate studies: A 1983 study (Hudson et al. 1983) found a kleptomania lifetime prevalence rate of 24% among a group of inpatient/outpatient/advertiser-responders with bulimia, and this statistic was then superimposed on a 1990 study (Whitaker et al. 1990) that found a 2.5% rate of bulimia among adolescents in a school district (Goldman 1991; Hudson et al. 1983; Whitaker et al. 1990). A more recent survey of ICDs in college students in 2010 found that although 27% had stolen at some point in his or her lifetime, the prevalence rate of kleptomania was 0.38% (Grant et al. 2010). This latter figure is likely more accurate because it was not dependent upon the diagnosis of an eating disorder.

Other samples have provided widely varying estimates of kleptomania: 4%–24% among shoplifters and 4%–9% among various psychiatric populations, including psychiatric inpatients, patients with alcohol use disorders, and depressed patients. Pathological gamblers have been found to have a 2%–5% rate of comorbid kleptomania (Grant 2006). In the Hudson et al. (1983) study on bulimia, a prevalence rate of 44% for kleptomania was found for patients with combined anorexia and bulimia; however, this was in a small sample of only 25 patients. Clearly, we have a lack of broadly sampled and unbiased epidemiologic data for kleptomania.

It has been estimated that the female to male ratio is 3:1 (Durst et al. 2001). The majority of case reports in the literature involve females, and the larger studies of patients with kleptomania have demonstrated a female predominance. Yet it has been suggested that perhaps females are more likely to present for psychiatric evaluation or to be referred for evaluation by the legal system, whereas male shoplifters are more likely to be sent to prison (Grant 2006).

Clinical Features

The key markers for the diagnosis of kleptomania are the irresistible and compulsive nature of the stealing, the increasing subjective sense of tension beforehand, and then the sense of relief or pleasure at the time of the theft. This is not stealing for personal gain but, rather, for relief of symptoms. It is done without the assistance of others. Individuals often feel guilty or depressed afterward, and the urge or craving to steal is often experienced as ego-dystonic. Individuals typically resist the impulse to steal and are aware that it is wrong, but urges and increasing tension lead to the compulsive behavior (American Psychiatric Association 2013). There is often an impulsive nature to the thefts as well, because they are not usually planned in advance. However, some individuals may report obsessive thoughts about stealing or progressive tension over a period of hours or days that precedes the theft (Grant 2006). The stolen items are usually unneeded, affordable, and of little value; one woman described frequently stealing multiple units of the same small shampoo bottles, yet going to a different store to buy a large bottle of the shampoo that she actually used (Grant and Kim 2003). The stolen items are usually thrown away, hoarded, surreptitiously returned, or given to someone else (Grant 2006).

Onset is typically in adolescence or early adulthood, but it can be as early as childhood or as delayed as late adulthood. There are few data to guide us on describing its course, but three "typical" patterns have been described: 1) sporadic, with brief episodes of kleptomanic behavior punctuating long periods of remission; 2) episodic, with relatively equal and protracted periods of kleptomanic behavior alternating with remission; and 3) chronic, with some degree of fluctuation in the behavior (American Psychiatric Association 2013). As mentioned in the "Discussion" section, there is often a significant delay (on the order of years) between onset of the behavior and clinical presentation; females tend to come to clinical attention earlier, in their mid-30s, whereas for males it may be some years later (Goldman 1991). Higher rates of kleptomania are found in adolescents and young adults compared with older adults, which has led some authors to speculate that the natural course of the disorder may be to "burn out" or remit with time. However, other studies have reported similar current and lifetime prevalence rates, suggesting a persistent and chronic course instead. Given that the vast majority of the data are gathered from clinical samples, we actually know very little about the natural course of kleptomania (Grant et al. 2010).

Individuals often avoid stealing if apprehension is likely, but they can become increasingly brazen, and the chance of apprehension is not always taken into account. Some individuals have described an increased thrill when there is a greater chance of being caught. A majority of patients also report that the value of stolen items increases over time, suggesting a form of tolerance (Grant 2006). Some studies have found that 64%–87% of individuals with kleptomania have been apprehended at some point. The majority steal from stores. Whereas the exact prevalence of shoplifting is not known, it has been estimated that $10 billion worth of items are stolen from retailers annually, and approximately 2 million Americans are charged with shoplifting each year (Grant 2006). Studies of shoplifters have found varied rates of kleptomania, from 4% to 24%, depending on the sample. If we assume a conservative estimate of 5% of shoplifters with kleptomania, this translates to 100,000 arrests and a $500 million loss each year due to the disorder (Aboujaoude et al. 2004).

Ordinary shoplifters are more likely to engage in stealing sporadically and for personal gain, and they are found to be younger compared with a group of people with kleptomania. The group with kleptomania reported a larger number of prior thefts (Grant 2006). The behavior can often continue despite multiple convictions for shoplifting, and there is a clearly a subset of individuals with kleptomania who will have repeated arrests and severe legal problems, with resulting social impairment (Presta et al. 2002).

Comorbidity appears to be the rule with kleptomania. Available data suggest a lifetime prevalence of comorbid affective disorders ranging from 45% to 100% and ranging from 60% to 80% for anxiety disorders; the rates tend toward the higher end when subsyndromal forms are included (Grant et al. 2010). Rates for comorbid obsessive-compulsive disorder (OCD) specifically have been widely variable, with some studies ranging from 0% to 6.5% and others ranging from 45% to 60% (Grant 2006). Rates of 23%–50% have been found for comorbid SUDs, with alcohol and nicotine being the most commonly used substances. Other ICDs, such as compulsive sexual behavior, compulsive buying, or skin picking, appear to be comorbid in 20%–46% of individuals with kleptomania (Grant et al. 2010). Trichotillomania and pathological gambling have also been found to have increased comorbidity, although they have both been relocated out of the ICD category (Grant and Kim 2002). Eating disorders are frequently seen, with varying estimates of 10%–44% in individuals with kleptomania; bulimia is more common than anorexia nervosa (Presta et al. 2002). Some authors have also noted an increased frequency of somatic illness and a low degree of socialization (Sarasalo et al. 1996).

It also appears that personality disorders are comorbid in kleptomania, with a rate of 43% in one study (Grant 2004). Paranoid, schizoid, and borderline personality disorders were the most frequently diagnosed personality disorders, although the first two have been removed as official disorders in DSM-5. In the earlier literature, it was noted that traits such as "compulsiveness, dependency, lability, hysteria and histrionics" were observed in those with kleptomania (Goldman 1991). Some reports suggest that individuals with kleptomania are more likely to have stressful childhoods, marital discord, and low self-esteem or to be socially isolated. In a family history study, individuals with kleptomania were more likely to have first-degree relatives with alcohol use disorders or any psychiatric disorder when compared to a control group (Grant et al. 2010).

One recent study by Odlaug et al. (2012) noted an alarmingly high rate of 24% for suicide attempts among adolescents and adults with kleptomania, which is higher than for major depressive disorder or panic disorder. Even more surprisingly, 92% of attempts were attributed to the kleptomania itself, indicating a high level of distress about these symptoms. Such attempts were correlated with comorbid bipolar disorder, other ICDs, and personality disorders (especially borderline and narcissistic personality disorders); interestingly, all of these syndromes share a neurobiological deficit of executive function, which is also true for kleptomania. Although anxiety, depression, and SUDs did not correlate with increased risk of suicide attempts (which is inconsistent with prior literature), the study authors noted that they did not include completed suicides, and so this group might have been underrepresented. Similarly, legal issues were not significantly correlated, but there are anecdotal reports of patients committing suicide after arrest or conviction. Other risk factors for suicide in patients with kleptomania include shame, poor self-esteem, high levels of impulsivity and disinhibition, and social isolation (Odlaug et al. 2012).

The case of Sherry demonstrates a number of these comorbidities: major depressive disorder, generalized anxiety disorder, bulimia, an alcohol use disorder, somatic illness, and social isolation along with marital discord. There is also a notable connection between her depressive symptoms and her kleptomanic behavior, and she describes intense urges and cravings similar to those found in SUDs. In the section "Etiology," we discuss the affective spectrum and addictive disorder models for kleptomania, which can help to explain the symptomatology observed in Sherry.

Etiology

So how can we characterize kleptomania? As described in the "Clinical Features" section, kleptomania has been categorized in DSM-III through DSM-5 as an

ICD. However, in the scientific literature, we have seen significant overlap with mood disorders and SUDs, and some authors have speculated that kleptomania can be classified as an "affective spectrum disorder" or an addictive disorder instead (Grant et al. 2010; McElroy et al. 1991). It has also been suggested that kleptomania is related to OCD or even attention-deficit/hyperactivity disorder (ADHD). Finally, there are a number of cases described in the literature in which kleptomanic behavior has been temporally linked to an organic deficit, such as a traumatic brain injury, epilepsy, or progressing dementia (Goldman 1991). In the end, it is likely that the behaviors we classify as kleptomania will turn out to be far more heterogeneous than originally suspected and with a variety of etiologies.

Yet before examining these modern conceptualizations of kleptomania, it can be helpful to look at the earlier work of the psychoanalytic community. As early as the 1920s, the dynamics underlying kleptomania were being discussed and debated in the literature. There was a general consensus that such behavior was the symptom of an underlying conflict and that depression or disturbed sexuality was often present as well. Because the objects are not stolen for their economic value, some authors have suggested that the theft is for "intrapsychic profit" (e.g., Goldman 1991). Otto Fenichel proposed that kleptomania represented the gratification of id impulses and was closely tied to infantile needs, whereas Abraham discussed its relation to feelings of neglect from childhood. Karl Abraham thought that such compulsive stealing was a way of regaining pleasure that was not attained in childhood and at the same time symbolically exacting a revenge (Goldman 1991).

On the other hand, early drive theorists posited that compulsive stealing performed a sexual function, because it was "doing a forbidden thing secretly" (Goldman 1991). There have been case reports of patients who have associated fetishistic behavior and patients who described sexual arousal at the time of stealing, but this is not a consistent feature in kleptomanic patients in general (Fishbain 1987). Object relations theorists were concerned with the internal representations of the stolen objects and felt that such stealing could be a way of controlling a frightening object and therefore feeling omnipotent. Indeed, some patients in case reports are described as having a sense of omnipotence (as demonstrated by stealing more brazenly), but this does not always appear to be conscious. Self theorists viewed kleptomania through the lens of structural deficits in the self and postulated that stealing helped to repair narcissistic injuries and prevent fragmentation of the self (Goldman 1991). Unfortunately, modern case reports rarely mention details that would allow psychoanalytic assessment, so it has not been possible to confirm or rule out these proposals about the underlying dynamics of kleptomania.

In terms of our modern-day conceptualization of kleptomania, the most helpful framework seems to be a psychiatric classification of the disorder. DSM-III through DSM-5 categorize kleptomania as an ICD. True to their name, ICDs have traditionally been characterized by impulsivity, although recently, there has been increasing recognition of aspects of compulsivity within these disorders as well. It is now becoming clear that impulsivity and compulsivity can co-occur or appear at different times within one disorder (Grant and Potenza 2006).

Impulsivity can be defined as a "predisposition toward rapid, unplanned reactions to either internal or external stimuli, without regard for negative consequences" (Grant and Potenza 2006, p. 540). Impulsivity is a feature of many disorders and not just ICDs, including SUDs, personality disorders, bipolar disorder, and ADHD. On the other hand, *compulsivity* is defined as "the performance of repetitive behaviors with the goal of reducing or preventing anxiety or distress, not to provide pleasure of gratification" (Grant and Potenza 2006, p. 540). Compulsivity can be found in a variety of disorders as well, including OCD, SUDs, and personality disorders.

It is clear that aspects of both impulsivity and compulsivity can characterize the behavior and feelings of someone with kleptomania, and the intensity of each varies per individual. Baylé et al. (2003) found that patients with kleptomania had higher impulsivity scores than comparison groups of psychiatric patients and patients with alcohol use disorders and that this impulsivity was the key marker in a psychopathological profile specific to kleptomania. The one neuroimaging study that has been conducted in patients with kleptomania revealed decreased white matter microstructural integrity in inferior (ventral-medial) frontal regions (Grant et al. 2006); similar deficits have also been noted in subjects with other impulsive behaviors. This area is crucial for executive functioning, so deficits here likely result in poor decision making and an inability to appropriately balance immediate reward and potential punishment (Grant 2006).

The group with kleptomania also had high sensation-seeking and disinhibition scores, similar to the patients with alcohol use disorders. Compulsivity is demonstrated in individuals with kleptomanic behavior by its repetitive nature and the increasing tension that is felt before a theft, so that the act of stealing acts to reduce anxiety and tension (even if it ultimately results in depression or shame). In one study, it was found that more than half of patients hoard the items they steal, which is also a behavior that could be classified on the compulsive spectrum (Grant and Potenza 2006).

Noting the high rates of comorbidity among patients with kleptomania, many researchers have postulated alternate conceptualizations of kleptomania that remove it entirely from the realm of ICDs.

Some proposed alternative models are discussed here.

Addictive Disorder Model

The addictive disorder model is particularly compelling because the phenomenology of kleptomania mirrors SUDs in many ways, and there is increasing research support for such a connection. Similar to SUDs, individuals with kleptomania 1) experience urges to engage in behaviors that have negative results, 2) feel increasing tension beforehand and while resisting such urges, 3) experience significant pleasure during the behavior (this is more true in the earlier stages of SUDs), 4) experience rapid yet temporary reduction in the urge after the behavior, 5) note the return of such urges within hours to weeks, 6) respond to triggers linked to external cues (particular locations or items, etc.), and 7) develop second-order conditioning linked to internal states (such as boredom, stress, dysphoria, etc.) (Grant 2006). Whereas many subjects with kleptomania could identify specific triggers for their urges, some described waking up in the morning with the urge to steal and were unable to pinpoint anything specific (Grant and Kim 2002). This has also been described in individuals with SUDs.

As mentioned in the section "Clinical Features," 23%–50% of patients with kleptomania have a comorbid SUD, most often alcohol or nicotine, and first-degree relatives of individuals with kleptomania have a higher rate of alcohol use disorder than the general population. Psychological testing has demonstrated high scores of impulsivity and sensation seeking, similar to the those with SUDs (Grant et al. 2010).

In addition, there are growing data about the neurobiological commonalities of kleptomania and SUDs. Serotonergic, dopaminergic, and opioidergic pathways all appear to play a role in kleptomania, and these same pathways are implicated in the behavioral addictions in general. Serotonergic dysfunction has been shown on the platelet serotonin transporter in one group with kleptomania, and increased cognitive impulsivity seen in more symptomatic individuals is thought to be partly mediated by the serotonin system. Regarding dopaminergic pathways, patients with Parkinson's disease who receive dopamine agonists have developed a range of impulsive/compulsive behaviors, including shoplifting.

The opioidergic system is thought to be involved in urge and craving regulation via gabaminergic interneurons, which influence dopamine neurons in the nucleus accumbens (the reward center). The opioid antagonist naltrexone was found to be effective in reducing kleptomanic behavior in a group of patients who experienced urges to steal, and this represents the only evidence-based pharmacotherapy for kleptomania that we have so far. Last, the neuroimaging study described earlier in which subjects with kleptomania were found to have decreased white matter integrity in inferior frontal regions turned out to be very similar to findings in a separate study of cocaine-dependent patients (Grant et al. 2010).

Obsessive-Compulsive Spectrum Model

Kleptomania is characterized by irresistible and uncontrollable impulses to steal, and resisting these impulses leads to anxiety and tension. Similarly, in

OCD, there is an irresistible drive to engage in excessive and unwanted rituals, combined with increasing anxiety if these rituals are not performed. However, co-occurrence studies of kleptomania and OCD have been inconsistent, with widely varying rates of OCD found in patients with kleptomania (from 0% to 60%). Kleptomania is found in patients with OCD, ranging from 1% to 5.9%, at higher rates than the general population. Yet family history studies have also been inconsistent, with the only controlled study failing to find a higher rate of OCD among first-degree relatives of subjects with kleptomania (Grant and Potenza 2006).

Neurobiological research may offer some clues about a potential connection. Similar dysfunction was found in the platelet serotonin transporter among subjects with OCD and those with kleptomania, and there are case reports of kleptomanic behavior developing after damage to the orbitofrontal-subcortical circuits. A shared effective treatment for the two disorders could also support the idea of similar biological underpinnings. Whereas there was initial excitement when positive responses with selective serotonin reuptake inhibitors (SSRIs) were seen in patients with kleptomania, subsequent case reports have been inconclusive about their effectiveness (Grant 2006). The only controlled trial for SSRIs to date was negative; escitalopram was found to be equivalent to placebo (Koran et al. 2007). However, perhaps some of these negative results are due to a lack of narrowing of the sample to patients with kleptomania who share features with OCD, and perhaps this is a group that might consistently benefit from SSRIs or other OCD-related interventions and treatment.

Other limitations of this model include the facts that many individuals with kleptomania describe an urge or craving prior to the act of stealing and that the behavior itself can be pleasurable—neither of which is seen in OCD. Also, people with OCD tend to be harm avoidant and compulsively risk averse, whereas individuals with kleptomania have been shown to be sensation seeking and disinhibited (Grant 2006).

Affective Spectrum Disorder Model

It has been proposed that the term "affective spectrum disorders" might encompass a variety of psychiatric disorders that respond to antidepressants without necessarily being mood disorders, and they might therefore have a shared underlying pathophysiological basis. These disorders include major depressive disorder, panic disorder, OCD, bulimia, migraine, irritable bowel syndrome, cataplexy, and ADHD hyperactive-impulsive type (Hudson and Pope 1990). It was subsequently suggested that kleptomania, likely along with all ICDs, might also fit into this category. McElroy et al. (1991) argued that there are several lines of evidence to suggest this: 1) the high comorbidity of anxiety and depressive symptoms in kleptomania, 2) reports of kleptomanic behavior alleviating depressive symptoms, 3) reports of resolved kleptomanic symptoms after treatment with antidepressants or electroconvulsive therapy (ECT), and 4) the association of kleptomania with eating disorders, which, in turn, are strongly related to mood disorders.

Although effective treatment with antidepressants has not turned out to be a consistent feature of kleptomania, markedly elevated rates of comorbid affective disorders have been demonstrated in the range of 45%–100%. Some authors have also described the mood-elevating effects of theft and noted that some individuals appeared to utilize kleptomanic behavior as a sort of antidepressant during periods of depressed mood. Some case reports described clearly alternating patterns of depression and impulsive-type behaviors (e.g., kleptomania, sexual compulsions, compulsive buying), with the onset of the impulsive-type behavior leading to relief of the depression (Baylé et al. 2003).

For example, there was a case of a 54-year-old woman who impulsively stole unneeded food items and found rapid, profound relief of the depressive and anxiety symptoms that had arisen during diazepam withdrawal; other cases described remission of major depressive symptoms during periods of active kleptomania and recurrence of depressive symptoms after apprehension and cessation of the behavior (McElroy et al. 1991). However, this pattern has mostly been demonstrated in reports of single cases and requires further study (Baylé et al. 2003).

Similar to the addictive disorder and obsessive-compulsive models, the affective spectrum disorder model appears to be compelling in a subset of patients and may prove to be another "type" of kleptomania.

Attention-Deficit/Hyperactivity Model

The attention-deficit/hyperactivity model is a relatively recent model that is still in its infancy. It was suggested after observing that some individuals with kleptomania appear to have an inattentive, impulsive drive to shoplift similar to symptomatology seen in ADHD, and there have been a few anecdotal reports of effectively using ADHD medications to treat kleptomanic symptoms in such patients. One study of kleptomanic patients found a lifetime prevalence of 15% for ADHD. This model requires further study.

Organic Model

New-onset kleptomania has been described in two cases of closed-head trauma, and there have been reported cases of epilepsy and frontotemporal dementia preceding the onset of kleptomania. In addition, kleptomania has been reported as a side effect of SSRIs in at least three patients (Talih 2011). Although clearly only applicable to a small subset of patients with kleptomania, it is important to keep in mind that organic brain injury can lead to such symptoms.

So how can we reconcile these different models of kleptomania? On the basis of research and clinical experience, Grant and Kim (2003) have proposed that kleptomania remain within the realm of ICDs. They have also proposed, however, that patients with kleptomania be categorized according to three distinct subtypes: 1) those whose behavior is driven by urges (approximately 50% of patients), 2) those who are driven by an emotional state, such as being bored, lonely, anxious, or sad (10% of patients), and 3) those who experience a combination of urges and emotions (40%). The first subtype is often triggered by external cues, and this type is clearly akin to the SUDs. The second type could be considered an affective spectrum disorder, yet the authors also pointed out that patients categorized within this subtype describe their behavior as an "escape" and that this can also resemble patients with SUDs who are experiencing relief craving. The third subtype is a mix of the first two, and patients in this category describe only feeling urges to steal when in certain emotional states, such as feeling lonely or sad. Our case of Sherry would probably fall into this third category (Grant and Kim 2003).

Further research needs to be done to verify these proposed subtypes and to investigate possible connections to OCD and ADHD. Organic etiologies of kleptomanic behavior can inform neurobiological research regarding specific affected brain regions.

Differential Diagnoses

Before diagnosing kleptomania, some other diagnoses and situations should be considered. Kleptomania needs to be distinguished from *ordinary theft,* in which the stealing is deliberate and motivated by the worth of the object—regardless of whether it is planned or impulsive. Sometimes theft may be an act of revenge or rebellion, undertaken "on a dare," or a rite of passage. In all of these cases, there would be a lack of the required symptomatology of kleptomania: compulsivity, tension leading up to the act, and relief or pleasure at the time of the act. Shoplifting and ordinary theft are common, whereas kleptomania is rare (American Psychiatric Association 2013).

Malingering needs to be ruled out. Some individuals may feign the symptoms of kleptomania in order to avoid criminal prosecution. Similarly, stealing in the context of conduct disorder and antisocial personality disorder is distinguished from kleptomania by an overall pattern of antisocial behavior. Stealing in the context of acute psychiatric or cognitive symptoms also needs to be regarded differently. Kleptomania is not diagnosed if the individual is stealing (either intentionally or inadvertently) during the course of a manic episode or if the stealing is in response to hallucinations or delusions during a psychotic episode. If the person is cognitively impaired as a result of a major neurocognitive disorder, the diagnosis of kleptomania is also not made (American Psychiatric Association 2013).

Treatment

Last, we look at how to engage the patient with kleptomania and various treatments that have been studied. Although this treatment research it still in its early stages, there have been some interesting findings.

How to Talk to Patients

The beginning of any discussion about a diagnosis of kleptomania should focus first on clarifying the diagnosis, including the exact nature and relative intensities of the symptoms experienced (e.g., urges vs. impulsivity vs. comorbid affective symptoms). This is crucial for treatment planning. A thorough interview should also include determination of specific comorbid disorders, including other ICDs, SUDs, affective disorders, OCD/anxiety disorders, eating disorders, and personality disorders. It is always essential to assess for suicidality and to perform a thorough risk assessment. It can be helpful to gather data about the time course of the kleptomanic symptoms as related to other mood symptomatology, because a mood-elevating effect of kleptomanic behavior has been proposed (Baylé et al. 2003).

Successful treatment of kleptomania, as with any other ICD, involves educating patients that they have an illness and that without treatment, the illness is likely to be lifelong (Grant and Kim 2003). Additionally, anticipatory guidance and subsequent psychotherapy should address the fact that for some individuals, the kleptomania has become a part of their identity and has at times enabled the them to feel good. This should not be ignored when assisting patients to develop new and more healthy coping skills to handle distress and, in fact, should be discussed throughout the course of treatment (Grant and Kim 2003).

Psychosocial and Pharmacological Treatments

At present, there are no manualized psychotherapeutic treatments for kleptomania, nor are there any medications approved by the U.S. Food and Drug Administration (Grant 2006). However, the literature includes examples of a wide variety of treatments for kleptomania, although to our knowledge there is only one randomized controlled trial to date that has demonstrated the efficacy of a psychopharmacological treatment (naltrexone) (Grant et al. 2009). A good deal of the literature about the treatment of kleptomania focuses on the models discussed (addictive disorder model, obsessive-compulsive spectrum model, affective spectrum disorder model, and attention-deficit/hyperactivity model), and treatment suggestions often stem from the evidence-based treatments for these respective disorders.

Psychosocial treatments in earlier decades used a psychoanalytic/dynamic approach in which the focus was on the "symbolic meaning... attributed to the act itself, the object stolen, and the victim of the theft" (Durst et al. 2001, p. 188). The psychoanalytic theories described earlier heavily influenced the therapeutic approach, depending upon the therapist's school of thought. In general, individual and group psychotherapy targeted at kleptomania has not shown sustained benefits when studied. More recently, cognitive-behavioral therapy has generated interest as a psychotherapeutic approach, although its efficacy in the treatment of kleptomania has not yet been empirically tested. Behavioral strategies include aversion therapy, covert sensitization (pairing imagery of the behavior with an unpleasant feeling and experiencing relief when imagining that the behavior ceases), systematic desensitization, and exposure and response prevention. Drawing on comparisons with the extensive literature on the treatment of OCD, some authors have suggested that even though it has not yet been systematically studied, it is likely that cognitive-behavioral therapy in combination with medication is more effective than medication alone (Durst et al. 2001).

As of now, there are no psychopharmacological treatments approved by the U.S. Food and Drug Administration that are available for the treatment of kleptomania. The literature on psychopharmacological treatments primarily consists of case reports and small, uncontrolled studies, although there has been at least one double-blind, placebo-controlled trial of escitalopram (Koran et al. 2007) and one of naltrexone (Grant et al. 2009). In these studies, only naltrexone demonstrated superiority to placebo. The literature on psychopharmacological treatments focuses on the following classes of medications: opioid antagonists, SSRIs, other antidepressants, and mood stabilizers. Case reports can be found pertaining to other agents as well, including atypical antipsychotics (aripiprazole), the catechol O-methyltransferase (COMT) inhibitor tolcapone, and even ECT.

Earlier, uncontrolled studies of naltrexone indicated it might be effective in treating kleptomania, and this has now been supported in a double-blind, placebo-controlled trial of naltrexone with doses ranging from 50 to 150 mg/day (mean effective dose 117 mg/day). Naltrexone demonstrated superiority over placebo. Subjects in this study were required to have had at least "moderate urges" to steal in the week prior to study entry, so this was a specific subset of patients with kleptomania. Naltrexone was hypothesized to exert its effect by decreasing dopaminergic neurotransmission in the nucleus accumbens via disinhibition of gabaminergic input to these dopamine neurons, thus reducing urges to steal and the subjective experience of pleasure (Grant et al. 2009).

There is arguably the most data about the use of SSRIs for the treatment of kleptomania, and it has been argued by some that SSRIs should be the first-line treatment because of the relatively greater numbers of case reports in the literature for these agents. It was expected that SSRIs would be effective in treating kleptomania, because they have been proven effective for trichotillomania and pathological gambling—which were also classified as ICDs up until the publication of DSM-5 (Durst et al. 2001). Fluoxetine is the SSRI most frequently cited as beneficial in kleptomania, although there are also reports of positive effects for fluvoxamine, paroxetine, and escitalopram. However, in the only double-blind, placebo-controlled trial of SSRIs for the treatment of kleptomania, Koran et al. (2007) found that "the high response rate during open-label escitalopram treatment was not better maintained by double-blind escitalopram than by placebo" (p. 426).

Other non-SSRI antidepressants have also been tried for the treatment of kleptomania, with case reports demonstrating positive treatment responses to trazodone, nortriptyline, and combinations of imipramine/fluoxetine, fluvoxamine/buspirone, and amitriptyline/perphenazine. Monoamine oxidase inhibitors have not been shown to be effective when used alone; there was just one case in which combining tranylcypromine and trazodone proved beneficial (Durst et al. 2001).

There are no controlled studies of mood stabilizers. Lithium, valproic acid, and topiramate have all been used for treatment of kleptomania. Lithium has not shown a convincing effect, with the few case reports in the literature showing mixed results, whereas the use of valproic acid is supported by at least two case reports (Durst et al. 2001). At least three case reports have shown topiramate to be helpful; this was postulated to involve the disinhibition of γ-aminobutyric acid in the nucleus accumbens (Dannon 2003).

In other categories of medications, there is at least one case report of aripiprazole being helpful in an individual with kleptomania that developed subsequent to a brain injury (Mercan et al. 2009), and Grant and Kim (2003) suggested that atypical antipsychotics may be useful in the treatment of ICDs in general. Likewise, one case report demonstrated effectiveness for tolcapone (a COMT inhibitor), and the authors speculated that it may enhance "cognitive functioning prefrontally resulting in greater inhibition of behavior and better decision-making regarding consequences of behavior" (Grant 2011, p. 295). As mentioned, the typical antipsychotic perphenazine was found to be helpful in one case when combined with amitriptyline. Clonazepam and alprazolam have been reported to show some success in reducing symptoms of kleptomania, and there are frequent anecdotal reports of using benzodiazepines to provide tension relief in the beginning stages of treatment. ECT has been beneficial in two published cases, but the effect may have been mediated through treatment of comorbid major depression (Durst et al. 2001).

Regarding which pharmacologic treatment to try first, opinions differ. Although SSRIs have most frequently been recommended as first-line treatment, there is now evidence that naltrexone is effective in the subset of patients who experience moderate urges to steal. Beyond this, there are few data to guide us. It seems that the best approach would be to identify the "subtype" of kleptomania for a particular patient (i.e., the associated symptomatology) and to use this information to choose an initial medication (Table 9–1). For patients with sig-

TABLE 9–1.   Pharmacological treatment strategies for kleptomania

Medication	Supporting data	When it may be most effective
Naltrexone	One RCT	Prominent urges/cravings to steal
SSRIs	Case reports (One RCT did not demonstrate efficacy of escitalopram over placebo.)	Comorbid affective disorder
Other antidepressants	Trazodone and nortriptyline have been shown to be effective in a few case reports.	Comorbid affective disorder
Mood stabilizers	Case reports	Comorbid affective disorder
Atypical antipsychotics	Case reports, anecdotal	Limited data
Psychostimulants	Anecdotal	Predominant impulsivity, comorbid ADHD

Note.   ADHD=attention-deficit/hyperactivity disorder; RCT=randomized controlled trial; SSRIs=selective serotonin reuptake inhibitors.

nificant mood or anxiety symptoms, antidepressants may be helpful; if manic symptoms or a bipolar diathesis is present, mood stabilizers should be considered. Patients who endorse urges/cravings to steal and/or a family history of SUDs should be given a trial of naltrexone. If kleptomanic symptoms appear to be within the context of the general impulsivity and inattentiveness seen in ADHD, psychostimulants can be considered (Grant 2006).

Resources in the Community for Treatment

There are also resources in the community, largely based on the 12-step model. For example, a Shoplifters Anonymous group in New York City defines itself on its Web site as a 12-step group for "compulsive shoplifters, stealers, thieves and kleptomaniacs." Groups under the names Compulsive Shoplifters Anonymous (CSA) and Cleptomaniacs and Shoplifters Anonymous (CASA) can also be found. Although there is little empirical evidence about the efficacy of these groups, recommending them in conjunction with medication and individual treatment is reasonable to consider (Grant and Kim 2003).

Key Points

- Kleptomania is likely rare, but it is underdiagnosed and can cause significant impairment legally and socially. Introduce the subject by normalizing the behavior to reduce shame, and then screen patients for it.

- Kleptomania is categorized as an impulse-control disorder, but there is also evidence that it may be an addictive disorder, on the obsessive-compulsive spectrum, or one of the "affective spectrum disorders." There are also cases of kleptomanic behavior beginning after organic injury. It is possible that kleptomania is a final common pathway for a heterogeneous group of etiologies.

- Naltrexone is the only evidence-based treatment for kleptomania at this time. Given the limited data, you should probably choose a treatment strategy based on comorbidities (see Table 9–1). Use opioid antagonists if craving or urges are prominent, antidepressants or mood stabilizers to target symptoms when there is a comorbid affective disorder, and psychostimulants if attention-deficit/hyperactivity disorder is present.

- Recent data suggest a high rate of suicide attempts in individuals with kleptomania (24%), with the overwhelming majority of attempts related to the kleptomanic behavior itself. These attempts were correlated with comorbid bipolar disorder, other impulse-control disorders, and borderline and narcissistic personality disorders. Make sure to assess suicidality in every patient with kleptomania and aggressively treat both the kleptomanic symptoms and any comorbid disorders.

References

Aboujaoude E, Gamel N, Koran LM: Overview of kleptomania and phenomenological description of 40 patients. Prim Care Companion J Clin Psychiatry 6(6):244–247, 2004 15614312

American Psychiatric Association: Diagnostic and Statistical Manual of Mental Disorders. Washington, DC, American Psychiatric Association, 1952

American Psychiatric Association: Diagnostic and Statistical Manual of Mental Disorders, 2nd Edition. Washington, DC, American Psychiatric Association, 1968

American Psychiatric Association: Diagnostic and Statistical Manual of Mental Disorders, 3rd Edition. Washington, DC, American Psychiatric Association, 1980

American Psychiatric Association: Diagnostic and Statistical Manual of Mental Disorders, 4th Edition, Text Revision. Washington, DC, American Psychiatric Association, 2000

American Psychiatric Association: Diagnostic and Statistical Manual of Mental Disorders, 5th Edition. Arlington, VA, American Psychiatric Association, 2013

Baylé FJ, Caci H, Millet B, et al: Psychopathology and comorbidity of psychiatric disorders in patients with kleptomania. Am J Psychiatry 160(8):1509–1513, 2003 12900315

Dannon PN: Topiramate for the treatment of kleptomania: a case series and review of the literature. Clin Neuropharmacol 26(1):1–4, 2003 12567156

Durst R, Katz G, Teitelbaum A, et al: Kleptomania: diagnosis and treatment options. CNS Drugs 15(3):185–195, 2001 11463127

Fishbain DA: Kleptomania as risk-taking behavior in response to depression. Am J Psychother 41(4):598–603, 1987 3434652

Goldman MJ: Kleptomania: making sense of the nonsensical. Am J Psychiatry 148(8):986–996, 1991 1853988

Grant JE: Co-occurrence of personality disorders in persons with kleptomania: a preliminary investigation. J Am Acad Psychiatry Law 32(4):395–398, 2004 15704625

Grant JE: Understanding and treating kleptomania: new models and new treatments. Isr J Psychiatry Relat Sci 43(2):81–87, 2006 16910369

Grant JE: Kleptomania treated with tolcapone, a catechol-O-methyl-transferase (COMT) inhibitor. Prog Neuropsychopharmacol Biol Psychiatry 35(1):295–296, 2011 21062636

Grant JE, Kim SW: Clinical characteristics and associated psychopathology of 22 patients with kleptomania. Compr Psychiatry 43(5):378–384, 2002 12216013

Grant JE, Kim SW: Stop Me Because I Can't Stop Myself: Taking Control of Impulsive Behavior. New York, McGraw-Hill, 2003

Grant JE, Potenza MN: Compulsive aspects of impulse-control disorders. Psychiatr Clin North Am 29(2):539–551, 2006 16650722

Grant JE, Correia S, Brennan-Krohn T: White matter integrity in kleptomania: a pilot study. Psychiatry Res 147(2-3):233–237, 2006 16956753

Grant JE, Kim SW, Odlaug BL: A double-blind, placebo-controlled study of the opiate antagonist, naltrexone, in the treatment of kleptomania. Biol Psychiatry 65(7):600–606, 2009 19217077

Grant JE, Odlaug BL, Kim SW: Kleptomania: clinical characteristics and relationship to substance use disorders. Am J Drug Alcohol Abuse 36(5):291–295, 2010 20575650

Hudson JI, Pope HG Jr: Affective spectrum disorder: does antidepressant response identify a family of disorders with a common pathophysiology? Am J Psychiatry 147(5):552–564, 1990 2183630

Hudson JI, Pope HG Jr Jonas JM Yurgelun-Todd D: Phenomenologic relationship of eating disorders to major affective disorder. Psychiatry Res 9(4):345–354, 1983 6580663

Juquelier P, Vinchon J: L'Histoire de la Kleptomanie. Rev Psychiatr Psycholog Exp 18:47–64, 1914

Koran LM, Aboujaoude EN, Gamel NN: Escitalopram treatment of kleptomania: an open-label trial followed by double-blind discontinuation. J Clin Psychiatry 68(3):422–427, 2007 17388713

Marazziti D, Mungai F, Giannotti D, et al: Kleptomania in impulse control disorders, obsessive-compulsive disorder, and bipolar spectrum disorder: clinical and therapeutic implications. Curr Psychiatry Rep 5(1):36–40, 2003 12686000

McElroy SL, Hudson JI, Pope HG, Keck PE: Kleptomania: clinical characteristics and associated psychopathology. Psychol Med 21(1):93–108, 1991 2047510

Mercan S, Karamustafalioglu OGUZ, Karabulut V, et al: Aripiprazole in the treatment of kleptomania: a case study. Eur Neuropsychopharmacol 19:S547–S548, 2009

Odlaug BL, Grant JE, Kim SW: Suicide attempts in 107 adolescents and adults with kleptomania. Arch Suicide Res 16(4):348–359, 2012 23137224

Presta S, Marazziti D, Dell'Osso L, et al: Kleptomania: clinical features and comorbidity in an Italian sample. Compr Psychiatry 43(1):7–12, 2002 11788913

Sarasalo E, Bergman B, Toth J: Personality traits and psychiatric and somatic morbidity among kleptomaniacs. Acta Psychiatr Scand 94(5):358–364, 1996 9124084

Talih FR: Kleptomania and potential exacerbating factors: a review and case report. Innov Clin Neurosci 8(10):35–39, 2011 22132369

Whitaker A, Johnson J, Shaffer D, et al: Uncommon troubles in young people: prevalence estimates of selected psychiatric disorders in a nonreferred adolescent population. Arch Gen Psychiatry 47(5):487–496, 1990 2331210

Questions

1.   Which of the following is NOT one of the DSM-5 criteria for kleptomania?

   A. Recurrent failure to resist impulses to steal objects that are not needed for personal use or for their monetary value.

   B. Increasing sense of relaxation and calmness immediately before committing the theft.

   C. Pleasure, gratification, or relief at the time of committing the theft.

   D. The stealing is not committed to express anger or vengeance and is not in response to a delusion or a hallucination.

   E. The stealing is not better explained by conduct disorder, a manic episode, or antisocial personality disorder.

The correct answer is B.

Criterion B for kleptomania in DSM-5 is "Increasing sense of tension immediately before committing the theft." The other criteria are correct as stated.

2. Which of the following classes of pharmacotherapy has been demonstrated in a randomized controlled trial to be effective for the treatment of kleptomania?

    A. Selective serotonin reuptake inhibitors (SSRIs).
    B. Mood stabilizers (lithium, valproic acid, topiramate).
    C. Opioid antagonists (naltrexone).
    D. Second-generation antipsychotics (aripiprazole, risperidone).
    E. Benzodiazepines (clonazepam, alprazolam).

The correct answer is C.

Although there are case reports and anecdotal evidence supporting pharmacotherapies of many types (including antidepressants, mood stabilizers, antipsychotics, and benzodiazepines), there has been only one randomized controlled trial that has demonstrated the efficacy of a pharmacotherapy for kleptomania. This trial showed that naltrexone at an average dose of 117 mg/day was superior to placebo in reducing stealing urges, stealing behavior, and scores on a kleptomania scale. The subjects included in this trial specifically endorsed feeling "moderate urges" to steal in the week prior to study entry.

3. Which of the following is TRUE regarding the epidemiology of kleptomania?

    A. The disorder is more prevalent in males than females, with an estimated 4:1 ratio of affected individuals.
    B. Broadly based, unbiased population data exist so that we can accurately estimate the comorbidity of kleptomania with other psychiatric conditions.
    C. Greater than 50% of shoplifters are thought to meet criteria for the diagnosis of kleptomania.
    D. There is thought to be high comorbidity (25%–50%) between kleptomania and substance use disorders.
    E. There is no evidence of an increased prevalence of eating disorders in individuals with kleptomania.

The correct answer is D.

The literature shows 23%–50% comorbidity of kleptomania with substance use disorders, with alcohol and nicotine being the most commonly abused substances. Kleptomania is thought to be more prevalent in women, with a 3:1 ratio compared to males. Broadly based, unbiased epidemiologic data regarding the prevalence of kleptomania and its comorbidites are lacking, although there are data to suggest a comorbidity with eating disorders as well (variably estimated at 10%–44%). Studies of shoplifters have found varied rates of kleptomania, from 4% to 24% depending upon the sample.

CHAPTER 10

Sex Addiction

The Fire Down Below

LISA J. COHEN, PH.D.

THERE is considerable agreement in the literature as to the existence of a condition characterized by driven and compulsive sexual behavior. Individuals with this condition can spend an inordinate amount of time pursuing essentially anonymous sexual encounters to the detriment of their personal life, occupational functioning, financial well-being, and even physical health. In the context of possible exposure to AIDS, such behavior can be life threatening. Certainly, the media is awash with sex scandals involving politicians who seemingly risk all they have achieved in the pursuit of repeated and largely anonymous sexual encounters; Eliot Spitzer and Anthony Weiner are only among the latest to sacrifice their careers on the altar of transient sexual gratification.

Nonetheless, there is considerable controversy in the literature as to how to conceptualize such behavior, and a variety of nomenclature has been proposed, including sexual addiction (Carnes 1991; Goodman 1998), hypersexual behavior (Kafka 2010), and paraphilia-related behavior (Stein et al. 2000). In this chapter, I present the case of a man with such driven, repetitive sexual behavior and then discuss the aspects of his presentation that reflect common features of sexually addictive behavior, as well as those components that may be unique to his history. The diagnostic considerations of driven and compulsive sexual behavior, particularly in light of the construct of sexual addictions, are reviewed. The possible neurobiological substrates of this condition are also considered, as well as treatment options.

The following is the case history of a man presenting in psychotherapy with sexually addictive behavior. This history represents a composite of several patients treated for sexual addiction in the past two decades. In order to preserve confidentiality, many of the inessential details have been changed, and components from multiple patients' histories have been incorporated into the story.

Clinical Case

Sam is a 42-year-old married man with two children. He was referred for psychotherapy at the request of his wife, who was concerned about his capacity to control his increasing urges for infidelity, which had precipitously increased after attending a party for his oldest child's seventh birthday. Although the patient was initially resistant to psychotherapy, he soon acknowledged that he was desperate to save his marriage and terrified at the thought of breaking up his family.

He reported a long history of polysubstance abuse (primarily involving alcohol, ecstasy, and cocaine), starting in his late teens and ending 2 years into his relationship with his wife, whom he met 10 years prior to entering treatment. With the exception of a few small relapses, he had easily remained sober since joining Alcoholics Anonymous (AA) 8 years previously. However, in the context of his substance abuse, he had chronically demonstrated compulsive sexual behavior, including promiscuous sex with women and some men, patronizing of prostitutes, and compulsive masturbation to pornography. As a young man in his 20s, he was a member of a fairly successful rock band and therefore had ample access to drugs and casual sex. Whereas discontinuing his drug abuse was relatively easy, refraining from compulsive sexual behavior was far more difficult. Although he later recognized an underlying shame at his out-of-control behavior, he had long seen his sexuality as ego-syntonic, a reflection of a free and honest spirit unconstrained by hypocritical societal conventions. He also viewed his sexual behavior as consistent with his philosophical opposition to monogamy.

In his early 30s, Sam met his future wife and wisely recognized this to be a relationship worth preserving. At this point, he joined AA, gave up substance abuse, and committed to living within the sexual parameters of his relationship. His wife agreed to sexual exploration at the outset of their relationship, including a few visits to sex clubs and one or two ménage à trois experiences with other women. After a while, however, Sam's wife became less accommodating to these activities, wondering why he was not satisfied with their sexual life together. Sam's sexual desire for his wife waxed and waned, along with his tolerance of intimacy with her. As treatment progressed and his comfort with intimacy and vulnerability with his wife increased, his sexual compulsivity decreased. However, during her business trips or when their children demanded more attention from her, Sam would develop intense new urges to visit a massage parlor, call a prostitute, or engage in anonymous sex with a woman he met in a casual encounter. He was relentlessly honest with his wife, but her tolerance of such confessions diminished over time, and such conversations grew increasingly painful for her.

At these moments, the ego-syntonic nature of these desires became increasingly prominent, and Sam's insistence on the normality and health of such behavior trumped his concern about his marriage. He insisted that he felt no need for the marriage, that such ties were artificial and overly burdensome, and that he could easily start again if he chose to simply walk away from the relationship. Interestingly, he spoke about his urge for sex with strangers as an uncomplicated desire for an intimate and honest encounter.

The entrenched nature of his sexual compulsivity reflected the young age at which Sam discovered the self-soothing properties of sexual stimulation. Sam was born in Tehran, the only son of a successful businessman with ties to the Shah's government. Sam's mother was the daughter of an English mother and an Iranian father; her father had also been wealthy and well connected. After the fall of the Shah's regime in 1979, the Sam's father felt it prudent to take his family out of the country and emigrate to Great Britain as soon as he could safely do so. When Sam's parents arrived in England in the 1980s, they found themselves in a far different environment than they had left. Although Sam's father found work in an engineering firm—drawing on his university education in engineering— his new position was an enormous step down from what he had before. His parents lost their elite status, their wealth, and their insider connections. They were exposed to racist attitudes that they had previously never encountered. From a comfortable place at the pinnacle of their society, they had fallen to the role of perpetual outsider. These narcissistic losses were most painful for Sam's father and led to distance between Sam's parents. Soon Sam's father embarked on a series of extramarital affairs. Sam's mother, who had been pampered and protected her whole life, was unprepared for these stresses on her family. Around this time, the family visited a beloved cousin, who was staying in a Swiss boarding school. Sam, missing his former companion, insisted that he wanted to join his cousin at boarding school. He was 7 years old at this time. Whereas sending children to boarding school was a time-honored tradition among the British upper classes and Swiss boarding schools had particular cachet, it is likely that Sam's mother found it convenient to send her child away so that she could devote herself more fully to her precarious marriage. It is unlikely that Sam's mother would have consciously entertained this thought, although it is certainly plausible that this could have been an unconscious incentive.

Although Sam adapted to boarding school over time, he spent the first year away from home crying himself to sleep, as did most of the children his age. Such naked displays of homesickness were cruelly mocked by the older boys, and Sam soon learned to suppress his emotions in general and his attachment needs in particular. Although his parents visited on holidays and his mother always showed great affection and happiness to see him, he experienced her visits as a demand that he turn his attachment to her on and off at what he perceived to be her convenience. He found this expectation deeply enraging and insulting, cementing a connection between attachment and humiliating powerlessness that would persist long into his adulthood. At around the age of 10, likely at the tutelage of older boys, he discovered the miraculous capacities of his penis and the emotional self-sufficiency afforded by masturbation. From this point on, he utilized masturbation as a potent means of self-soothing and an effective tool to banish homesickness and calm himself to sleep.

In his middle teens, the Sam began to engage in sexual activity with girls and a few homosexual encounters with classmates. In his late teens, he joined a rock band, which achieved surprising success in the following 2 years. He toured with the band for the next 10 years, fully embracing the sex, drugs, and rock-and-roll lifestyle now readily available to him, until the band broke up when he was 30 years old. This left him at loose ends until he met his future wife 2 years later. Although he effectively settled into a new life with his wife and growing family, a powerful resurgence of urges to engage in sexually addictive behavior occurred when his oldest child turned 7, the same age at which he first separated from his family.

Video 5 provides a dramatization of a therapy session with Sam. Notice how the patient alternates between seeing his sexual behavior as problematic and as personally acceptable. Notice also the personal meaning the behavior has for this particular patient. For this patient, the sexual behavior serves a self-soothing function in the context of perceived abandonment. Whereas the compulsive sexual behavior may be quite similar in different patients, the personal meaning ascribed to it may be unique to the patient's life history.

 Video Illustration 5: Addressing motivation to change in sexual addiction (5:23)

Discussion

Sam's case is instructive as it shows the intimate connection between regulation of negative affect and driven sexual behavior. Even though sexual outlets give him pleasure, he feels most compelled to pursue anonymous sexual contacts in order to master the negative emotions associated with abandonment. These urges are so compelling for him that he will risk the possible dissolution of his family. It is also important to consider the interpersonal meaning that his sexually addictive behavior has for him. He discovered masturbation as a child when forced to live separately from his parents, wrenched away from the soothing presence of his mother. In search of a means to self-soothe in the absence of maternal comfort, he discovered that sexual stimulation could serve that function for him, at least in part. In this way, sexual orgasm became fused with both the need for attachment and the ability to master that need, to be perfectly self-sufficient. Although sexual addiction does not always develop in this way and may not always fulfill this function, it is typical that an addiction can grow into the primary attachment for the addict. The commitment and attachment to the drug (or behavioral addiction) can displace any other relationship. As is not typical for many addicts, however, Sam is fairly able to control his behavior— that is, once he is motivated to do so. When he wants to stop, he can. However, his sexually addictive behavior is enabled by his rationalizations and other cognitive distortions. Because of this, Sam's therapy focuses less on developing skills for controlling his impulses and more on untangling his cognitive distortions and helping him identify his ultimate goals and priorities and recognize how such behavior will interfere with having the life he wants to have.

Diagnostic Considerations

As mentioned in the introduction, there is a fair amount of controversy over the construct of sexual addiction. Although this discussion can become somewhat technical, it is important to consider diagnostic issues because it helps clarify the nature of our patients' driven sexual behavior and therefore helps us to design effective interventions. Dating back to DSM-III (American Psychiatric Association 1980), repetitive, driven, and maladaptive sexual behavior has been classified as some form of sexual disorder not otherwise specified in the "Psychosexual Disorders" section of the manual. Importantly, such behavior does not involve an abnormal object of sexual arousal, as with paraphilias such as exhibitionism, voyeurism, and pedophilia, but, instead, it involves the excessive practice of otherwise normal sexual behavior. In 1991, Carnes observed that patients with such driven, repetitive sexual behavior showed many parallels with those who had chemical addictions. Carnes (1991) proposed the diagnosis of sexual addictions as a behavioral analogue of chemical addictions. He noted that the DSM criteria for substance dependence (DSM-III-R [American Psychiatric Association 1987] at that point) could be directly adapted to diagnosing sexual addiction. Carnes described a pattern of out-of-control sexual behavior that 1) interfered with social, occupational, and role functioning, 2) persisted despite negative consequences, 3) served to regulate negative affect states, and 4) persisted despite awareness of the need for and/or unsuccessful attempts to stop or reduce the behavior. These criteria are highly consistent with descriptions of similar sexual conditions and are therefore relatively noncontroversial (Goodman 1998; Kafka 2010). However, the next two criteria, tolerance and withdrawal, are less widely accepted and remain in need of further research. Carnes suggested that individuals with sexual addiction meet criteria for *tolerance*, characterized by pursuit of increasing levels of sexual activity over time as the prior levels no longer satisfy the individual's urges. Second, sexual addiction is characterized by *withdrawal*, such that the cessation of the sexual activity leads to emotional discomfort and dysphoria, a psychological if not physiological withdrawal syndrome.

Goodman (1998) further developed the concept of sexual addiction and elaborated on therapeutic interventions adapted from the treatment of chemical addictions.

More recently, Kafka (2010) specified the construct of hypersexual behavior in preparation for possible inclusion in DSM-5 (American Psychiatric Association 2013). In his diagnostic criteria, hypersexual behavior is characterized by a period of 6 months of recurrent and intense sexual fantasies, urges, or sexual behaviors in the context of three of the following five criteria: 1) excessive, time-consuming sexual activity interfering with other important goals, 2) repetitive engagement in such sexual activity as a means to regulate negative mood states,

3) repetitive engagement in such activity in response to stressful life events, 4) repeated but unsuccessful attempts to control such activity, and/or 5) continuing the activity while disregarding the risk for physical or emotional harm to self or others. Additionally, there must be clinically significant distress or impairment as a result of such activity, and the sexual activity must not be solely a result of a chemical substance. Although he did not specify the frequency of sexual activity in his diagnostic criteria, Kafka also proposed that seven sexual outlets (i.e., orgasms) per week marked a cut point for excessive sexual activity, based on his review of relevant research. Ultimately, the DSM-5 task force decided there were insufficient data to support inclusion of hypersexual disorder in the manual. We can see that Kafka's definition of hypersexual behavior significantly overlaps with Carnes' and Goodman's constructs of sexual addiction. Importantly, however, Kafka does not include the notion of tolerance and withdrawal, and he does not use the term sexual addiction as such.

Stein et al. (2000) discussed three models of maladaptive repetitive behavior through which to view "paraphilias not otherwise specified": impulsivity, compulsivity, and addiction. Although this chapter is focused on an addictive model of driven sexual behavior, it is useful to consider other possible approaches because they all have clinical implications. Compulsive behavior is driven by negative reinforcement and serves to decrease anxiety. The ideation is harm avoidant with an exaggeration of the likelihood of harm. A classic example involves patients with obsessive-compulsive disorder who compulsively wash their hands in order to reduce the anxiety occasioned by an obsessive fear of contamination. Sexual obsessions, in which the person is plagued by anxiety-inducing thoughts about the possibility of forbidden sexual urges and performs a compulsive behavior to reduce such anxiety, would fall into this category. In these cases, there is actually very little likelihood of the patient acting on the obsessive thought; rather, the problem derives from the patient's excessive concern about the possibility of harmful action.

In contrast, impulsive behavior is motivated by positive reinforcement and is characterized by the failure to inhibit pleasurable behavior despite negative consequences. There is inadequate thought about harmful consequences. People with sexual impulsivity are very likely to act on their sexual urges and are at high risk of behaving in reckless ways. Sexual impulsivity differs from sexually addictive behavior, however, in that the individual is only at risk of reckless behavior when tempted. Importantly, the primary problem is *inhibitory failure* rather than the strength of the urge.

Like impulsive behavior, addictive behavior is also motivated by positive reinforcement. As distinct from impulsive behavior, in which the inhibitory failure is the primary problem, in addictive behavior the *strength of the drive* is the primary problem. Nonetheless, addictive behavior is often driven by the need to reduce negative affect rather than by the pursuit of pleasure alone. In many cases, the addictive behavior starts out as pleasurable (positive reinforcement) but over time shifts so that it is driven more by the need to alleviate painful cravings (negative reinforcement) than to seek out pleasure per se (Kafka 2010). In either case, the strength of the desire is the cardinal problem, overwhelming the capacity for self-control. Keep in mind, however, that many patients with addictive problems also have problems with impulsivity.

Despite differences across these various approaches, there are numerous areas of overlap in descriptions of what might be called sexually addictive behavior. In all cases, there is 1) excessive sexual behavior, generally outside the context of sustained intimate relationships; 2) intense and persistent urges to perform such sexual behavior, similar to the drug craving found in chemical addictions; 3) continuation of sexual behavior despite the potential to cause significant harm with regard to personal, occupational, and financial domains and/or physical health; and 4) difficulty stopping the behavior despite repeated attempts or in the face of significant negative consequences. The presence of withdrawal or tolerance remains unclear.

In Sam's case, his sexual behavior is best characterized as addictive. It produces pleasure, is used to manage negative affect, and continues despite potential harmful consequences. Although he had fairly good control over his behavior by the time he was in therapy, in the past this was not the case. Importantly, he did not experience marked impulsivity across the board; Sam employed denial and rationalization when his urge to act overwhelmed his motivation to inhibit the behavior.

Neurobiological Substrates

Recent years have brought huge advances in our understanding of the underlying biology of addictions. Interestingly, the same dopaminergic tracts seem to underlie all types of addictions, both chemical and behavioral. Findings from animal and human research have pointed to the centrality of the dopaminergic reward circuitry, which courses from the ventral tegmental area in the midbrain through the nucleus accumbens in the striatal system. This system serves as an all-purpose motivation machine, active in all motivated pursuits and implicated in all disorders of reward-driven behavior (e.g., pathological gambling, binge eating, compulsive spending, sexual addictions). Although there are fewer data on behavioral addictions, we know that chemical addictions dysregulate the reward system and in extreme circumstances lead to significant deterioration of dopamine function in these tracts, leaving the individual that much more dependent on external sources of dopamine stimulation, such as cocaine and methamphetamine (Panksepp and Biven 2012; Volkow et al. 1999). According to a study by Garavan et al. (2000), the addiction may co-opt the reward system, so that other sources of reward no longer activate it as strongly as do cues related to the addictive object. This can explain how addicts of any type can sacrifice so much of what is truly important to them in pursuit of their addiction.

Whereas the dopaminergic reward system can explain the appetitive drive behind sexual addiction, it cannot explain the object of the addiction. Why does someone become addicted to sex rather than some other object or activity? With regard to sexually addictive behavior, premature sexual stimulation seems to play a key role. In particular, childhood sexual abuse may predispose individuals toward sexually dysregulated behavior. There is robust evidence that sexual abuse histories are disproportionately represented in individuals with pedophilia and other paraphilias (Cohen et al. 2010a; Kafka and Prentky 1997). Therefore, it is likely that people with sexually addictive behavior may also have a disproportionately high rate of childhood sexual abuse histories.

This is relevant to Sam's case as well. Although he did not experience childhood sexual abuse per se, in that no one coerced him to engage in sexual activity, he did engage in repeated sexual stimulation several years before he reached puberty. It has been proposed that premature sexual stimulation can alter sexual neurodevelopment (Cohen et al. 2010a). Two strains of evidence support this hypothesis. As mentioned, there is robust evidence of elevated rates of childhood sexual abuse in patients with pedophilia and other sexual disorders, in fact, considerably more than in patients with chemical addictions (Cohen et al. 2010a). Moreover, animal studies have shown that damage to neurobiological substrates of the sexual behavioral system differentially impacts sexual functioning, depending on the existence of prior sexual experience (Panksepp and Biven 2012). For example, lesions in the hypothalamus (anterior hypothalamus for males, ventromedial hypothalamus for females) will completely eliminate sexual behavior in rats if the lesions are created prior to sexual maturity. If the rat has already reached sexual maturity and already had sexual experience, however, the same lesions will have much less of an impact. This is seen to reflect the recruitment of higher-order cortical structures involved with learning and memory following the onset of actual sexual experience (see Panksepp and Biven 2012 for a review). Thus we could hypothesize that to the extent such findings can be generalized to humans, early sexual experience may alter the development of higher-order cortical regulation of sexual desire and behavior. Certainly, there is a failure of inhibitory mechanisms associated with frontal control in sexually addictive behavior. Likewise, the frequent demonstration of executive dysfunction among individuals with chemical addictions as well those with disordered sexual behavior is consistent with this hypothesis (Cohen et al. 2010b).

Treatment

Controversy remains about the diagnostic classification of driven and repetitive sexual behavior; however, there is less controversy about treatment, and multiple treatment options are currently available. Such options include individual psychotherapy, group psychotherapy, and psychotropic medication. The options for individual psychotherapy are particularly rich, and multiple modalities are available to address different components of the sexually addictive behavior (see Table 10–1).

Individual Psychotherapy

Cognitive-behavioral therapy (CBT) can address the mechanism of the addictive behavior, identifying and ultimately changing the thoughts, emotions, and behaviors that perpetuate the problematic behavior. More specifically, CBT can help the individual identify and better attend to the triggers of the sexually addictive behavior, the permission-giving thoughts that weaken inhibition of the behavior, and the negative consequences of the behavior. Specific modes of CBT that have been developed to treat chemical addictions have been modified to treat sexually addictive behavior (Carnes 1991; Goodman 1998).

Motivational interviewing is often used with chemical addictions and serves to help the patient consider the pros and cons of maintaining the addiction in the context of their overall goals and priorities (Miller and Rollnick 1991). Motivational interviewing is aimed less at actually changing the behavior than in shoring up motivation to enter the change process. The advantage of this approach is its nonconfrontational and nondirective nature, which is seen to be more effective with those patients with low motivation to change.

Although there is less research to support psychodynamic treatment in the field of addictions, it certainly offers advantages (Goodman, 1998). Specifically, psychodynamic treatment can address the factors related to the individual's unique personal history and personality organization. It can clarify the specific meaning the addictive behavior holds for the patient. Does sexual addiction reflect a rebellion against a puritanical and authoritarian parent? Is it a form of self-soothing in the context of parental abandonment, as with Sam? Does it assuage a narcissistic need for constant affirmation of one's attractiveness? Or is it used in a desperate attempt to stave off feelings of emptiness? In almost all cases, however, sexually addictive behavior reflects a disturbance in the core self-concept and/or the capacity for intimate relationships. As deeply social animals with lifelong attachment needs, it is inherent in the human condition to need close intimate relationships, which serve to regulate both negative and positive emotions (Mitchell, 1988; Panksepp and Biven 2012). Consequently, we are doomed to feel dependent on people who remain, in large part, outside

TABLE 10–1. Treatment options for sexual addiction

	Targets of treatment: problems with	Mechanisms	Disadvantages
Psychotherapy			
Cognitive-behavioral therapy	Behavioral control, management of negative affect, social skills, relapse prevention	Functional analysis of sequence and triggers of behavior, thought records, skill building	Does not address motivation, personal meaning, or underlying character structure
Psychodynamic	Self-concept and interpersonal relationships, self-awareness, underlying personality organization	Exploration of personal meaning of symptoms in context of personal history	Does not provide concrete skills to change behavior
Group	Shame, stigma, social isolation, denial, rationalization	Social support, group confrontation of denial, peer sharing of experiences	Does not provide individualized, in-depth treatment
Medication			
Treatments for comorbid conditions	Comorbid anxiety; depression, obsessive-compulsive disorder, impulsivity, psychosis, or mania	Established treatments of comorbid conditions can reduce symptoms of sexual addiction	Works best if sexual addiction secondary to or strongly exacerbated by comorbid condition
SSRIs	Anxiety, depression, obsessional ideation, sex drive	Reduces dysphoric affect, may reduce sex drive	Largely safe, but SSRIs not without side effects
Antiandrogens	Overall sex drive	Greatly reduces or eliminates sex drive	Severe side effects, including pulmonary embolism, bone mineral loss

Note. SSRIs=selective serotonin reuptake inhibitors.

of our control. For those who have less tolerance for this dilemma, often as a result of a maladaptive early attachment experiences, an addictive object can provide a convenient end run around the vulnerability and relative powerless inherent in intimate relationships with other people. In this way, sexually addictive behavior can serve as a sort of transitional object, a construct introduced by the British psychoanalyst D.W. Winnicott in the twentieth century (Winnicott 1965). Like the classic example of a toddler's baby blanket, sexually addictive behavior serves as a self-soothing and emotionally regulating "other" who, nonetheless, remains under the individual's almost total control. The sexual partners encountered in sexually addictive behavior are rarely experienced as "subjects"—three-dimensional people who can make an emotional impact on the sexually addictive individual outside of his or her control. Rather, they are fleeting "objects," used to gratify an urge and then discarded. Paradoxically, however, by insisting on total control over the attachment object, the sexually addictive individual actually loses control and ends up living at the mercy of his or her addiction. Psychodynamic therapy can help the patient to understand how these dynamics play out in his or her life and subsequently to develop healthier relational patterns.

In Sam's treatment, we used relatively few CBT techniques, because he had fairly good control over his behavior when he was motivated to control it. At the times during which he was at risk of acting on his sexual urges, the problem was more one of motivation than of impulse control. His behavior had become ego-syntonic, and he saw his sexual desires as in line with his values. At that point, motivational interviewing techniques often came into play, helping Sam to question his priorities and goals and to consider the extent to which his sexually addictive behavior helped or hindered him in reaching his life goals. Additionally, psychodynamic exploration aimed to improve his insight into his own emotional life.

Group Psychotherapy

Group treatment has been highly effective in the treatment of chemical and other behavioral addictions, and in some cases it is more effective than individual therapy alone (Goodman 1998). Group therapy serves multiple purposes and probably works through a combination of mechanisms. More specifically, group therapy provides social support for the difficult change process, information about other group members' experiences and coping strategies, support for a positive new group identity, and confrontation of the all-too-common denial and rationalizations associated with addictive behavior.

Twelve-step programs constitute a specific form of group therapy, the first and best known being AA. These are member-led groups composed of people with similar addictions who are committed to helping each other achieve and maintain sobriety. The 12 steps refer to a specific therapeutic plan to acknowl-edge the extent of the addiction and powerlessness over the addiction, to make amends for past behavior, and to commit to a lifetime of usefulness to other peo-ple. Since the first incarnation of AA in the early 20th century, a plethora of new 12-step programs have arisen, adapted for such problems as pathological gam-bling (Gamblers Anonymous) and overeating (Overeaters Anonymous). A number of 12-step programs for people with sexually addictive behavior are also available, including Sex Addicts Anonymous, Sexual Recovery Anony-mous, and Sex and Love Addicts Anonymous.

Sam briefly attended a 12-step program to become free from drug and alco-hol dependence. He found this helpful but was able to maintain sobriety without continued attendance within about a year. He did not attend a 12-step program for sex addiction, however, because he did not consistently identify himself as having this problem.

Medication

Although medication is not the first-line treatment for sexually addictive behav-ior, psychotropic medications are available for the treatment of such problems (see Thibaut 2012 for a review). To the extent that the problematic behavior is an outgrowth of or exacerbated by other psychiatric problems, such as mania, depression, anxiety, affective lability, and general impulsivity, medications shown to be efficacious with these conditions, such as mood stabilizers, antide-pressants, antianxiety medications, and second-generation antipsychotics, may be indicated.

Selective serotonin reuptake inhibitors (SSRIs) have also been investigated for their specific efficacy with sexually disordered behavior, but data from con-trolled trials are lacking. SSRIs may work to reduce compulsive thoughts be-cause of their antiobsessional effects. Additionally, the otherwise undesirable side effect of reduced sexual drive and function might be considered beneficial for individuals with hypersexuality.

When sexually disordered behavior offers grave risk to the individual or to so-ciety, for example, as in the case of persistent and uncontrolled pedophilia, antian-drogen therapy has been found effective in drastically reducing sexual drive. The side effects with this class of medication are notable, however, so it is unlikely that such medication will be used except in very grave circumstances. More recent treatments include gonadotropin-releasing hormone analogues, including leupro-relin and triptorelin, which provide a more advantageous side effect profile than older antiandrogen medications. Still, significant problems with bone mineral loss suggest the use of these medications is indicated only in high-risk situations.

Owing to ongoing depression and anxiety, Sam was treated with an SSRI to very good effect. This led to overall improvement in all areas of his mental health, including reduced interest in sexually addictive behavior. In this case, it is likely that his improvement was due to effective treatment of the comorbid mood and anxiety problems rather than of his sexual inclinations per se.

Conclusion

Excessive sexual behavior is a relatively common and often highly problematic condition. A behavioral addiction model provides a useful framework for conceptualizing and treating both the common features and the unique aspects of a patient presenting with sexually addictive behavior. Key factors for the clinician to keep in mind when evaluating such patients involve the patient's 1) motivation to change, 2) level of impulse control, and 3) personal meaning that the behavior may have for the patient. Cognitive-behavioral, psychodynamic, and group therapy as well as various medications all provide useful treatment strategies; these should be employed according to the needs of the individual patient.

Key Points

- Although there is controversy over the construct of sexual addiction per se, there is general agreement about a condition characterized by repetitive, out-of-control, and driven sexual behavior, typically conducted with strangers, which leads to distress or dysfunction.

- Whereas the sexual encounter itself may be experienced as pleasurable, the sexually addictive behavior generally serves to manage and control negative affect.

- Patients with this condition can show poor insight into the problematic nature of their behavior, using elaborate rationalizations to justify it.

References

American Psychiatric Association: Diagnostic and Statistical Manual of Mental Disorders, 3rd Edition. Washington, DC, American Psychiatric Association, 1980

American Psychiatric Association: Diagnostic and Statistical Manual of Mental Disorders, 3rd Edition, Revised. Washington, DC, American Psychiatric Association, 1987

American Psychiatric Association: Diagnostic and Statistical Manual of Mental Disorders, 5th Edition. Arlington, VA, American Psychiatric Association, 2013

Carnes P: Don't Call It Love: Recovery from Sexual Addiction. New York, Bantam, 1991

Cohen LJ, Forman H, Steinfeld M, et al: Comparison of childhood sexual histories in subjects with pedophilia or opiate addiction and healthy controls: is childhood sexual abuse a risk factor for addictions? J Psychiatr Pract 16(6):394–404, 2010a 21107144

Cohen LJ, Nesci C, Steinfeld M, et al: Investigating the relationship between sexual and chemical addictions by comparing executive function in subjects with pedophilia or opiate addiction and healthy controls. J Psychiatr Pract 16(6):405–412, 2010b 21107145

Garavan H, Pankiewicz J, Bloom A, et al: Cue-induced cocaine craving: neuroanatomical specificity for drug users and drug stimuli. Am J Psychiatry 157(11):1789–1798, 2000 11058476

Goodman A: Sexual Addiction: An Integrated Approach. Madison, CT, International Universities Press, 1998

Kafka MP: Hypersexual disorder: a proposed diagnosis for DSM-V. Arch Sex Behav 39(2):377–400, 2010 19937105

Kafka MP, Prentky RA: Compulsive sexual behavior characteristics. Am J Psychiatry 154(11):1632, 1997 9356590

Miller WR, Rollnick S: Motivational Interviewing: Preparing People for Change. New York, Guilford, 1991

Mitchell SA: Relational Concepts in Psychoanalysis. Cambridge, MA, Harvard University Press, 1988

Panksepp J, Biven L: Archaeology of Mind: Neuroevolutionary Origins of Human Emotions. New York, WW Norton, 2012

Stein DJ, Black DW, Pienaar W: Sexual disorders not otherwise specified: compulsive, addictive, or impulsive? CNS Spectr 5(1):60–64, 2000 18311101

Thibaut F: Pharmacological treatment of paraphilias. Isr J Psychiatry Relat Sci 49(4):297–305, 2012 23585467

Volkow ND, Wang GJ, Fowler JS, et al: Association of methylphenidate-induced craving with changes in right striato-orbitofrontal metabolism in cocaine abusers: implications in addiction. Am J Psychiatry 156(1):19–26, 1999 9892293

Winnicott DW: The Maturational Processes and the Facilitating Environment. New York, International Universities Press, 1965

Questions

1. Withdrawal and tolerance are

    A. Always found in patients with sexual addiction.
    B. Well documented in the literature.
    C. Physiological responses to the cessation of sexually addictive behavior.
    D. A point of contention among researchers, who disagree on whether repetitive, driven sexual behavior should be called an addiction.

    The correct answer is D.

Originally, sexually addicted behavior was proposed as a direct analogue of chemical addiction, including the presence of tolerance and withdrawal. This means that individuals with sexual addiction would require more sexual outlets over time (tolerance) and that on stopping the behavior, the person would feel anxiety, dysphoria, or some other type of psychological withdrawal reaction. It was not suggested that the withdrawal would be physiological, as with a chemical addiction. This has been the most controversial part of the notion of sexual addiction, because there is, to date, very little evidence either for or against the presence of tolerance and withdrawal.

2.   Group therapy CANNOT help with which of the following?

   A. Providing social support and reducing stigma.
   B. Combating denial and rationalizations.
   C. Providing a new, positive social identity.
   D. Providing in-depth understanding of one's personality organization.

The correct answer is D.

Group therapy is a powerful method of supporting change. It harnesses the power of group dynamics to help participants create a new positive identity, based on their membership in a group of people committed to mastering their addictions. Likewise, this type of therapy helps reduce stigma and isolation, as group members share their experiences and struggles with one another. Because all group members have experienced problems with addiction, they are well equipped to recognize and confront rationalization and denial in other group members, and they can do so without alienating or shaming the person in question. Group therapy does not, however, afford the opportunity for in-depth analysis of the individual's history and personality structure. That must be done in individual therapy.

3.   Cognitive-behavioral therapy (CBT) is LEAST useful in the treatment of

   A. Poor impulse control.
   B. Relapse prevention.
   C. Lack of motivation to change.
   D. Poor communication skills.

The correct answer is C.

CBT focuses on the mechanics of behavioral change. It identifies the thoughts and behaviors that perpetuate the problematic behavior and emotions and suggests alternative, more adaptive strategies. In this way, CBT is very effective with improving impulse control and communication skills as well as enhancing relapse prevention. CBT only works, however, if the person is already motivated to change and shares the same goals for treatment with the therapist. Because motivation to change is such a cardinal issue in any kind of addiction, alternative modalities, such as motivational interviewing, may be needed if the person lacks sufficient motivation to make effective use of CBT.

CHAPTER 11

Love Addiction

What's Love Got to Do With It?

Alexis Briggie, Ph.D.
Clifford Briggie, Psy.D., LADC, LCSW

LOVE addiction, the term initially proposed for this chapter, enjoys widespread endorsement from addiction therapists and the recovery community. Outside the recovery world, therapists are familiar with the dynamics and issues of these patients, but therapists tend to conceptualize them within the framework of attachment disorder, borderline personality disorder, separation anxiety disorder, and posttraumatic stress disorder. Support from therapists has, nevertheless, been growing, albeit with some reluctance. Much of the acceptance by the behavioral health field at large is driven by advances in understanding the neuroscience of addiction; media reports about celebrities with sex and other addictions and the resulting popular support of the concept; and the large number of people who self-identify as love addicts.

Love addiction has also been imprecisely defined and inconsistently applied, reflecting conceptual confusion and raising doubts about both the term and the nature of the disorder. Among many alternative terms are attachment disorder (Bowlby 1988), codependence (Beattie 1986), maladaptive romantic love (Hartney 2013), women who love too much (Norwood 1979), dependent personality disorder (American Psychiatric Association 2013), borderline personality disorder (American Psychiatric Association 2013), relationship dependency (Moore 2010), separation anxiety disorder (American Psychiatric Association 2013), relationship obsession (Moore 2010), and romantic obsession (The Augustine Fellowship 1990).

Defining the Addiction

We can start to sort out the plethora of perspectives by looking at healthy, mature love. Genuine love expresses itself through empathy, caring, and nurturing emotions and behavior. Its energy is affirming and compassionate. Healthy love cannot be an addiction, just as an addiction cannot be healthy love. Hence the term "love addiction" makes little sense. In addition, some of the contradictory elements of love addiction (and its variants) led us to think that there might be more than one type. (A comparison of healthy and unhealthy relationships can be found in Table 11–1.)

In search of a more accurate term, we looked closely at exactly what it is that is *craved* by individuals who are in romantic relationships and who self-identify as love addicts. We received two answers to our question: 1) One group craves the *euphoric high* of new romance, and 2) the other group craves the *security* of a relationship that will last "forever." In addition, this latter group also has high hopes—and strong expectations—that their *lives will be transformed* by this partner, erasing past trauma or other attachment disasters and making them happy. The dialectic of transformation and security is striking but beyond the scope of this introduction. These two types of craving correspond exactly to the two phases—*attraction* and *attachment*—of healthy love. Attraction and attachment also represent the normal progression of healthy love in a romantic relationship. Developmental failures such as insecure attachments, traumatic loss and separation, failure to thrive, interrupted (or absent) bonding, physical and psychological neglect, and maternal mental illness (including postpartum depression and psychosis) can distort that progression. The result of attachment failure is a multitude of problems with love and relationships. Love becomes compulsive, obsessive, addictive, and dependent, and remains immature. It is love gone awry; it is the experience of self-identified love addicts.

We now use the term *romantic relationship addiction*, defined as the maladaptive craving for, and pursuit of, romantic relationships to experience a euphoric high or powerful sense of security and worth that will tranquilize one's loneliness and related affective distress. Craving and pursuit continues despite causing harm and negative consequences. Loss of control, tolerance, and withdrawal also develop. Two subtypes—*attraction phase* and *attachment phase*—refer to the phase of the relationship that the patient most craves.

Attraction Phase

In the attraction phase of this addiction, the craving is for the euphoria of a romantic encounter. This is your brain on romance. The individual feels high, the result of changes in the brain and, in turn, changes in mood, cognition, and behavior. The smitten individual experiences a dizzying array of emotions best

TABLE 11–1. Healthy and addictive romantic relationships: a comparison

Healthy romantic relationship	Addictive romantic relationship
Emotional clarity and intimacy	Emotional intensity, a romantic high
Desire for true intimacy and commitment	Fear of true intimacy and commitment
Development of relationship over time, working on problems	Instant love, leaving at first sign of trouble
Ability to focus on the rest of life	Serious distraction by romantic obsession/fantasy
Loyalty and commitment	Moving to next relationship quickly, always searching
Satisfied and satiated	Lonely, empty, dissatisfied, cannot get enough
Ending of maladaptive relationships	Doing anything for partner to stay
Mutual support	Contingent support, controlling
Acceptance and support of partner's autonomy	Jealous of anything that competes with "our time"
Ability to trust	Distrust and suspicion, fear of trusting
Realistic expectations	Extreme, unrealistic expectations: romance will "cure" problems and provide meaning to life
Confidence in partner's return, enjoys solitude	Fear of abandonment, cannot be alone
Honesty	Lying to preserve the relationship
Openness, friend and confidante with partner	Secrecy, hiding true feelings from partner
Compatibility required	Emotional attachment without knowing person
Improvement of each partner's life in relationship	Deterioration of personal life for one or both partners

TABLE 11–1.　Healthy and addictive romantic relationships: a comparison *(continued)*

Healthy romantic relationship	Addictive romantic relationship
Confident commitment, able to trust partner	Frequent reassurance needed, will test loyalty and monitor partner, makes frequent demands
Recognition that mindless or self-defeating love is not healthy	Sacrifice of financial stability, reputation, and self-respect for love
Integration of relationship with rest of life, not cut off	Isolation of self and partner
Acceptance of each other's weakness, support of strengths	Idealization at the beginning, devaluation at the end
Healthy use of boundaries and limits	Progressive loss of control, no effective boundaries or limits, even as relationship gets more destructive

characterized as expansive, exciting, and pleasurable. The intoxication of this phase is what people call falling in love, limerence, or infatuation (not unlike the first love of adolescence).

The attraction phase of romantic love is a healthy, normal process and is enjoyed equally whether one is addicted to it or not. Most people experience it as a very intense, sometimes delightfully impulsive and zany, period in a new romantic relationship. Suddenly, the world looks different. We are experiencing an altered state of consciousness. Our mood is labile: we feel joyful and euphoric when we think about or spend time with our lover and sad and a little empty when we part from, or long for, our lover. We obsess about our new love interest and want to be with him or her as much as we can. We attribute "all things wonderful" to him or her. We are restless; our sleep, appetite, and energy change. Our sexual appetite is awakened and on full alert. When young and infatuated, we feel invincible; when older and infatuated, we feel young again.

Individuals with compulsive attraction are not concerned with sustaining a relationship. They are solely concerned with obtaining and repeating the high of initial, idealized love. When the high starts to fade, or ends, they will typically and quickly "jump ship" and start a new romantic relationship. They truly believe that the next relationship will be different. In a *non*addictive relationship, this same moment would mark the transition from attraction to attachment.

Attachment Phase

In the attachment phase of romantic relationship addiction, the craving is for a sense of security and continuity in a relationship. The individual is far less interested in the fireworks of new romance and is almost solely interested in sustaining the relationship. Their enjoyment of the attraction phase is often, in fact, much less pleasurable than it appears. Enjoyment may even be feigned as an investment in eventual attachment and long-term bonding with their love interest. Many of those with compulsive attachment have been traumatized in their early years and may have a very difficult time tolerating, let alone enjoying, their partners' (for example) phase-appropriate wish for frequent sex.

Attachment theory focuses on how early relationships develop when they are "shaped by threat and the need for security" (Holmes 1996; see also Bowlby 1988). Later on, when remaining in a maladaptive adult relationship "because I love him/her," it is clear that the individual who makes that statement does not know what healthy love is. Attachment becomes pathological when the individual will do anything—like tolerate domestic violence, affairs, verbal and emotional abuse, theft, and substance abuse—to keep the relationship together. They may regard their lovers' outburst of pathological jealousy as a demonstration of their partners' love. Troubled attachment or trauma in childhood strongly *predisposes* or *primes* individuals to repeat these compulsive attachment patterns throughout the rest of their lives.

Attachment is also a normal, healthy process that follows the initial period of attraction. Healthy attachment, however, is very different from compulsive attachment. As the passion storms of attraction start to die down from their greatest intensity, attachment becomes more important and persistent. Deep and powerful feelings of empathy, caring, commitment, and concern for the lover's well-being now emerge. The ultimate success of attachment is long-term bonding, which continues to mature over a lifetime. Healthy attachment is most strongly determined by having had healthy models of attachment and not having been exposed too much to adverse childhood experiences. It also develops as the partners' develop more sober knowledge about each other as real people rather than as love-struck idealizations. It is, in one sense, a falling *out* of love with one's imagined ideal lover and falling *in* love with a real person. Healthy attachment is not devoid of conflict, dependency, and neurosis. All relationships, no matter how healthy or positive, contain at least some elements of unhealthy dependency and attachment.

For those with compulsive attachment, the search for secure and loving attachment becomes wrapped up in any and every new relationship. Unerringly, they choose partners who are unable to express authentic intimacy. There is an expectation that security (attachment) will follow the initial attraction. But hope and expectation evaporate as the initial infatuation loses intensity and attachment does not follow. Despondency, emptiness, and self-loathing—an all-pervading feeling of being bereft—emerge in the vacuum. Despite the severity of such pain (and other negative consequences), the individual obsesses about and compulsively repeats the same pattern, truly believing that next time, things will work out well.

The attachment phase addict is unable—despite his or her best efforts—to maintain a relationship with a healthy individual. Their internal template of healthy intimate relationships is simply too damaged and distorted to do so. Individuals who are attachment driven and have endured exposures to sexual victimization may be unable to enjoy the euphoria of a new relationship. They become overwhelmed with fear, and if they feel unable to express their distress to their lover, they are left trying to simply bear the touch and sexual intimacy. They may dissociate, use substances to numb themselves, or repeat thoughts to try to convince themselves that this is an acceptable investment in future attachment. Their emotional state is often overrun with flashbacks of sexual trauma and panic. Finally, both subtypes tend to exhibit some confusion about love, need, sex, and dependence. They tend, analogously, to funnel stress, guilt, loneliness, anger, shame, fear, and envy into longing and sexuality. The psychodynamic factors and addiction dynamics are intertwined and must be treated together.

Is Romantic Relationship Addiction *Really* an Addiction?

The American Society of Addiction Medicine, in their new definition of addiction (Smith 2012), no longer talks about chemicals, behaviors, and relationships but instead talks about the brain. Having a shared, common biological basis for addiction provides a platform to understand and accept the existence of addictions that are not yet widely accepted. The definition of *addiction* of the American Society of Addiction Medicine begins as follows:

> Addiction is a primary, chronic disease of brain reward, motivation, memory and related circuitry. Dysfunction in these circuits leads to characteristic biological, social, psychological, and spiritual manifestations. This is reflected in an individual's pathological pursuit of reward and/or relief by substance use and other behaviors. (Smith 2012, p. 1)

More and more research is confirming that chemical and neuroanatomical processes involved in addiction are similar regardless of the type of addiction (e.g., Burkett and Young 2012; Fisher et al. 2010). Functional magnetic resonance imaging has shown that pathological gamblers playing the slots show the same brain patterns as chemical addicts using crack cocaine (Potenza 2008). It also shows how phases of romantic love compare with images of individuals with chemical addiction (Fisher et al. 2010).

Romantic relationship addiction is like any other substance use disorder in DSM-5 (American Psychiatric Association 2013). The following criteria have close to unanimous acceptance for the diagnosis of addiction and apply to chemical, behavioral, and relationship addictions (a comparative chart is provided in Table 11–2): 1) Repeated use of a chemical, behavior, or relationship causes harm or suffering or impairs one's ability to meet adult role requirements (as father, partner, etc.). 2) Use is continued despite negative consequences (with work, money, relationships, legal issues [fights, arrests, driving under the influence], physical health, self-esteem, self-respect, feelings of shame). 3) More and more difficulty stopping the behavior is experienced. The initial euphoric promise of use starts to fade as 4) need and craving become more pronounced, and as 5) control over the addiction increasingly falters. The chemical, behavior, or relationship becomes increasingly central in the addict's life until it becomes a single-minded pursuit more important than anything else. 6) Pleasure gives way to need as escalating use becomes necessary to get the same effect (tolerance), and 7) highly distressing physical and psychological responses to loss of the drug or relationship (withdrawal) close in on the addict. The progression of addiction is accompanied by desperation, shame, ever-decreasing hope, and near total loss of behavioral control when it comes to the chemical, behavior, or relationship.

TABLE 11–2. Substance and romantic relationship addiction: a diagnostic comparison

Diagnostic feature	Substance addiction	Romantic relationship addiction
Recurrent behavior leading to significant impairment or distress	X	X
Recurrent behavior despite negative consequences/role impairment, e.g., at work, school, or home and with parenting, legal, social, and primary relations	X	X
Loss of control: ability to discontinue behavior increasingly difficult to exert. Rationalizations are attempted to give person the illusion of control ("I never drink before noon." "I lost my job because I wanted to see my boyfriend. I wanted a new job anyway.")	X	X
Tolerance: need for an increased dose to get the same effect ("Prove to me that you really love me. Stop seeing your friends.")	X	X
Withdrawal: acute, distressing symptoms experienced upon discontinuation of the substance or behavior	X	X

The nature of romantic relationship addiction may be further illuminated by the characteristics we expect to see in someone who recovers from it. Those characteristics include, among others, realistic expectations of what a relationship can and cannot provide; capacity to develop an independent identity, serious interests, and meaningful personal relationships (whether or not the individual is in a romantic relationship); autonomy; belief in one's own individual value; honesty; trust; and the ability to establish and maintain personal limits and boundaries.

Clinical Case

Jenny is a 24-year-old, unemployed single woman who presents for psychotherapy in the context of a breakup with her boyfriend. She was self-referred after a 28-day stay at an inpatient rehabilitation center, where she was treated for opiate dependence and codependence. It is noteworthy that although her parents were paying for her treatment, they were otherwise not involved; she has been estranged from them for several years prior, reconnecting with them only after a 1-year relationship with her boyfriend came to a chaotic end.

Although Jenny entered treatment of her own accord, she presents as distant, aloof, and moderately dissociated. Her presentation is much more consistent with that of someone being forced into treatment against her will; she is slow to warm up and does not become affectively engaged or connected until several months into the treatment. There is a marked contrast between her compulsion to make immediate connections with the men she engages with in her romantic relationship addiction dynamic and her initial, distant presentation with her therapist. The connection she does make is much slower and is punctuated later by sudden departure without direct discussion with her therapist.

Jenny reports a long history of polysubstance abuse, including alcohol, cocaine, heroin, ecstasy, and marijuana, beginning at age 13, which is significant because it is the same age she identifies as entering puberty and becoming interested in boys. She grew up in an affluent suburb and attended private school, where she had significant social difficulties throughout elementary and middle school. She describes being teased, particularly by other girls, causing her to seek out relationships with boys and older kids outside of school. She describes her substance use at that time as helping her feel connected to the boys she spent time with. She used drugs exclusively when with them (i.e., she never used alone) and provided them with substances and/or money for substances as a way to keep them close.

Jenny describes her father as overly strict, distant, and hyperlogical, and she describes her mother as both intrusive and absent. She felt it was difficult to get her parents' attention, and when they did pay attention, they were punitive and reprimanding. At an early age, she learned to suppress her needs for attachment and emotional closeness with family and to seek it outside of her family. The parental dynamics of alternating deprivation and intrusiveness left her hungry for genuine intimacy, which she attempted to find through the substitute gratification of both drugs and maladaptive relationships with men.

In 11th grade, Jenny dropped out of high school to run away from home with an older boy named Jim from her hometown, saying this was due to her parents being too "rigid and controlling" and her being "totally in love" with Jim. She described feeling consumed by thoughts of Jim, uninterested in anything else and willing to give up anything to stay in the relationship. She, in fact, gave up the physical safety and security of her home in order to hitchhike across the country with Jim, often enduring periods of homelessness and not having money to eat. She was also almost constantly drinking and/or smoking marijuana at this time, simply seeing it as something that she and Jim "liked to do together."

Throughout her teens and early 20s, Jenny continued a pattern of intense, brief relationships with men who physically and/or emotionally abused her. She would relocate to a new city only to move in with another version of the man she had left behind. When relaying her history throughout the course of treatment, she very clearly defined herself by these relationships and used them as a way to organize her sense of self and time. She never graduated from high school and never held a job, and she had seemingly little awareness about the connection between this and her preoccupation with relationships.

Jenny's most recent relationship before entering treatment was with a man named Alex, a moderately famous musician. They primarily used opiates together, which she said made her feel happy, in love, and close to him. When Alex was on tour or at work during the day, Jenny would use stimulants or "whatever she could find" in order to distract herself from the painful feelings of emptiness that she experienced during separations from him. When Alex ultimately left her, saying she was "too clingy," her substance use increased dramatically along with her feelings of loss, loneliness, and emptiness. She initially refused to leave the apartment they shared, isolating herself for days at a time, calling him repeatedly to try to convince him to change his mind, and sending long, pleading text messages. When Alex took out a restraining order against her, Jenny checked herself into an inpatient rehabilitation center.

When Jenny left inpatient treatment and transitioned to outpatient psychotherapy, she moved back in with her parents. Here she became reacquainted with the familiar feelings of her childhood and young adulthood, because her needs for attachment and connection were once again met with distance and rejection. In an attempt to feel better, she started going to Alcoholics Anonymous (AA) and Sex and Love Addicts Anonymous (SLAA) meetings, which were suggested by her therapist at her inpatient treatment program. After a few days of going to both meetings, she stopped attending SLAA meetings. She continued going to AA meetings, where she said she reconnected with George, an old friend from high school. Jenny strongly and repeatedly expressed that George was just a friend and that she was determined to keep it that way. She said was afraid of becoming "codependent," having learned this terminology in rehab; Jenny tried to create rules for herself in an attempt to guard against dependency.

She speaks often of her fear of becoming codependent and talks longingly about meeting the right guy who will cure her of this. She consciously tries to set boundaries in her relationship with George. She tries to set a weekly quota for reaching out to women (as opposed to men) for fellowship after meetings; she sets limits about how many days per week she allows George to drive her to and from meetings; she sets limits about how often she can spend time with him in general; she vows to never have sex with him. She also creates elaborate justifications about why she specifically needs George to drive her (e.g., she doesn't want to be a burden to her parents, her house is on his way, etc.) and generally rationalizes that the relationship is necessary because she no longer has any friends in her hometown.

When Jenny shares her fears of becoming too dependent with George, he begins to pull away. In response to this, Jenny begins to feel desperate to "win him back," ultimately offering to have sex with him via text message as a way to entice him to spend time with her even though she is not sexually attracted to him. She is unable to tolerate the distance he imposes between them (and her increasing feelings of abandonment), and in the meantime, Jenny reaches out to old boyfriends to spend time with her, attempting similarly to entice them with drugs and/or sex.

Shortly thereafter, Jenny abruptly terminates treatment without informing or discussing it with her therapist, who later learns that Jenny has checked herself into an inpatient rehabilitation center for the second time.

Discussion

As a child, Jenny had normal needs for love, safety, caregiver reliability, consistent attention, affection, encouragement, nurturance, affirmation, and validation. The alternating rhythm of parental neglect and intrusion, and of emotional coldness and shaming, that she experienced did not meet these needs. It left her feeling inadequate, defective, and unworthy. She had little, if any, self-confidence or positive self-regard. She believed, with her very young and still-developing brain, that if the people who are supposed to love you do things that hurt or feel bad to you, then you must be bad, defective, and undeserving. Jenny was unable to imagine that her parents' ability to provide healthy love was impaired. She learned at an early age to suppress her needs for attachment and emotional closeness within her family, because an adequate response from them was not forthcoming. She continued to look outward to fulfill her developmental needs, ultimately seeking this outside of her family.

In her early attempts to find nurturing outside of her family—in school—she was teased by other girls. In what must have felt like another failed environment, she sought relationships with boys and older kids outside of school. The use of drugs and her ability to get money to purchase them seemed to help her social life initially, but it was an illusory improvement. With her hunger for genuine intimacy and her fear that she was truly unacceptable, she began to seek acceptance for who she could be for others, further weakening her own identity and alienating herself from her true self. Without a foundational experience affirming her as a lovable, worthwhile individual, she was left with drugs and maladaptive relationships with men. Both were substitute gratifications, and both were inadequate.

Jenny's relationships have been attraction driven. She focused on this euphoric phase of romantic relationships to relieve—to tranquilize—her sense of rejection, loneliness, and emptiness. Urges and cravings for a romantic high are associated with poor partner choice because who the chosen person is does not really matter. The feeling is all that counts. The analogy can be made to polysubstance dependence, in which the addict will indiscriminately take any drug that is available to get high or numb. So, too, with Jenny: she would risk just about anything to maintain the high.

Jenny's substance and relationship addictions, as well as her separation anxiety, are intertwined. Her radar for tracking cooling interest or passion in her lover is supersensitive and, when detected, raises her anxiety to the level of panic. She experienced a lack of affection, intimacy, and structure in her development, and she has been in search of it ever since. Chemicals and relationships were a means to self-soothe, avoid, or numb herself in the absence of affection, intimacy, and structure and in the absence of other alternatives. She did not develop skills to soothe herself, and she found with chemicals at least some temporary respite. Compared with her parents' neglect and the rapid turnover of men in her life, alcohol and drugs became loyal, reliable companions to her, and, like a "best friend," they always got the job done.

Jenny's resilience and authentic self are also evident. She has survived, her perseverance is strong, and she retains awareness of her genuine, true self. That nascent self had been knocked down, but not out, more than once. Following her failed attempts to recover her sense of self through drug use and overly dependent, compulsive relationships with men, she finally sought treatment. During these several episodes of care, she began to develop insight into the connections between her childhood experiences, her problems with attachment, and her substance abuse. She began to attend 12-step meetings and attempted to set limits in relationships. Her recovery remains a work in progress.

Diagnostic Considerations

Romantic relationship addiction would be our primary diagnosis of choice for this patient were it included in DSM-5. However, the new definition of addiction of the American Society of Addiction Medicine (Smith 2012) boldly focuses on the neurobiological foundations of chemical and behavioral addictions rather than focusing on the specific chemical or behavior. This provides compelling support and legitimacy for the diagnosis and bodes well for inclusion of additional behavioral addictions in DSM in the near future.

Posttraumatic stress disorder should be investigated further. Jenny revealed a pattern of repeated relationships in her late teens and 20s in which she was physically and emotionally abused. There is no mention of childhood physical abuse, but clearly there was neglect. Abuse, coupled with her manifestation of dissociation in treatment, suggests that further exploration of posttraumatic stress could be quite useful.

Borderline personality disorder should be a diagnostic consideration because of Jenny's fear of abandonment, stormy interpersonal relationships, and impulsive substance abuse. Her identity disturbance is demonstrated by the fact that her interests and behaviors have been chosen according to what her lovers found appealing or what she thought would endear her to them, not for her own development. She felt that she was not accepted for whom she really was, so Jenny worked on becoming accepted for what others wanted.

The best available diagnosis, in lieu of love addiction or romantic relationship addiction, is *separation anxiety disorder*, a disorder that involves a "developmentally inappropriate and excessive fear or anxiety concerning separation from those to whom the individual is attached" (American Psychiatric Association 2013, p. 190). Jenny meets the requisite number of diagnostic criteria, including 1) "recurrent excessive distress when anticipating or experiencing separation from…major attachment figures"; 2) "persistent and excessive worry about losing major attachment figures "; and 3) "persistent and excessive fear of or reluctance about being alone or without major attachment figures" (American Psychiatric Association 2013, pp. 190–191).

Finally, Jenny's history is significant for abusing alcohol, cocaine, cannabis, heroin, and ecstasy. Drug use has been, for her, "a way to connect." She would use "whatever she could find" in order to distract herself from the painful feelings of emptiness that she experienced when separated from her compulsive love relationships. Her use of substances has always been secondary to her compulsion for attachment and fear of separation. Nevertheless, Jenny meets DSM-5 diagnostic criteria for all of the drugs mentioned—that is, alcohol use disorder, cocaine use disorder, cannabis use disorder, heroin use disorder, and ecstasy use disorder.

Treatment

See Video 6 for a dramatization of a clinical encounter that exemplifies how the here-and-now relationship between patient and therapist can be used to facilitate insight into the patient's relationships with others. In the treatment of love addiction, as the therapeutic alliance deepens, the relationship can be an incredibly powerful therapeutic tool to promote insight and effect change.

 Video Illustration 6: Power of therapeutic alliance (6:20)

Several elements are important independent of which approaches are used with Jenny: 1) a strong therapeutic alliance; 2) regular monitoring of the here-and-now relationship between patient and clinician; 3) a therapist who is aware and comfortable with obsessive, compulsive, dependent, and addictive elements in his or her own personality; and 4) direction without judgment or confrontation. Jenny's behavior represents her best current effort and skill for coping, symptom management, impulse control, and self-soothing. The plan would be to enhance the positive coping skills that Jenny already has while expanding her repertoire of new skills. Her developmental deficits, especially those having to do with attachment, also require therapeutic work. Jenny has separation anxiety, romantic relationship addiction, and substance use disorders. The standard for treating these is to combine cognitive-behavioral therapies (individual or group), individual psychodynamic psychotherapy, and self-help groups.

Talking With Patients About Compulsion, Attachment, and Addiction

The conversation with patients about compulsion, attachment, and addiction should always start with getting enough information about a patient that the clinician can mirror the patient's language and use terms that the patient feels most at ease with. What does "romantic relationship addiction" mean to the patient? What language feels most comfortable? Is there another term that feels more fitting for that person? How has this problem manifested itself in his or her life, and how has it interfered? How has it changed over time? For example, Jenny's involvement in addiction treatment 12-step groups provides a shared language for discussion.

Psychobehavioral Approaches

"Techniques are what you do until the therapist gets there" (C. A. Whitaker, personal communication, University of Connecticut School of Medicine, September 1975). So get there. Before any techniques—old standards or exotic new ones—are employed, put down your pen and move out from behind your desk and away from the computer and electronic medical record. Sit facing your patient with nothing in the way. Look at him or her. Make contact. Find out who this person is. Find out what is motivating him or her and what he or she *really* wants from treatment. Remain aware of how he or she affects your gut. When you have done that, you can use almost any technique, but do not lose sight of how you started. In psychotherapy, it is the relationship that heals.

Psychodynamic Psychotherapy
Psychodynamic psychotherapy expands a patient's awareness and insight. The therapist sparks and encourages the patient's curiosity about the origins and dynamics of his or her thoughts, emotions, and behavior. Unconscious dynamics and influences are exposed to scrutiny, especially how they express in the external world of the patient's interpersonal life and in the therapeutic relationship.

Some of Jenny's difficulties resulting from her compromised development include the following: anger about her parents' neglect of her; overwhelming feelings of loneliness, emptiness, inadequacy, and unworthiness; perception of others as part-objects; and self-loathing. These issues are responsive to psychodynamic psychotherapy.

Cognitive-Behavioral Therapy

Cognitive-behavioral therapy (CBT) and CBT-related therapies can help individuals identify distortions and errors in thinking and mistaken, irrational beliefs that underpin current maladaptive functioning. Patients learn to identify these distortions by, among other things, monitoring their internal dialogue (e.g., "you can't do that," "don't even try") and remembering childhood pronouncements (e.g., "you'll never amount to anything," "you're lazy and stupid") that compromise current functioning. Assessing the validity of patients' conclusions and considering different ways to view themselves and their capabilities are both potent CBT interventions. Finally, through role playing or in vivo exposure, they can experiment with alternative views and behaviors. CBT-based approaches also teach coping skills, symptom management, relapse prevention (for addictions), impulse control, and anger management.

Dialectical Behavioral Therapy

Dialectical behavioral therapy provides an atmosphere of validation coupled with psychoeducation and training in practical coping skills. The skills are core competencies for human life—skills that ordinarily would have been learned growing up in a healthy family. There are four primary skill sets:

1. Mindfulness helps patients cultivate present moment awareness. This enables them to observe and describe what is actually occurring without judgment. It is an antidote to seeing a new romance through the lens of their distorted hopes, expectations, and past beliefs about lovers. For many patients who say they miss their childhood/family/lover, what they really miss is what they wish it had been, not what it actually was.
2. Emotion regulation helps relationship addicts to not overreact in the face of emotions that threaten to overwhelm them. They become more aware of their feelings and the precursors to losing emotional control. Patients are taught how to downregulate those states of arousal, relieving the pressure for impulsive behavior. Upregulation is also taught, so that the individual does not ignore faintly recognized but painful reactions alerting them that something is not right in the relationship.
3. Distress tolerance helps patients learn multiple methods of tolerating distress without having to resort to self-defeating or self-destructive behavior. One such method—when experiencing acute relationship-related anxiety

or distress—involves self-soothing by engaging the five senses. For example, you can *listen* to or sing a favorite song; *watch* a travel video of a beautiful location; savor the *taste* of a favorite food; light a candle with a favorite *smell*; and *touch* or rub some soft material or a smooth stone. Jenny could have used these or other methods—such as taking a bubble bath, going for a run, buying herself flowers, or watching an engaging television show—to help tolerate her feelings of emptiness and loss in the wake of her breakup with Alex.

4. Interpersonal effectiveness helps patients learn a repertoire of skills that allow them to improve what have typically been stormy, volatile relationships. In this module, patients learn skills related to, among other things, self-respect, assertiveness, inhibition of emotions, limit setting, and setting and maintaining personal boundaries. Interpersonal effectiveness also provides psychoeducation about commonly held relationship myths and encourages the patient to begin to dismantle maladaptive beliefs by coming up with challenge statements (see Table 11–3).

Motivational Interviewing

Motivational interviewing is a systematic, evidence-based approach to complex behavior change. It is unique in eliciting and exploring patients' own arguments for change, evoking intrinsic motivation, and helping the patient to resolve his or her ambivalence about change (Miller and Rollnick 2002). Motivational interviewing is a directive but nonconfrontational method, bypassing unproductive struggles. The therapist engages the patient through empathic listening, open-ended questions, reflective statements, affirmations, and summary statements. This method decreases denial and enhances motivation. It is a very pragmatic, practical approach focused on actual change. For Jenny, it can provide psychological space for her to make her own decisions.

Group Psychotherapy

Group psychotherapy is the treatment of choice for a number of disorders, including chemical, behavioral, and relationship addictions. Therapists who do not practice group therapy sometimes consider it superficial compared with individual therapy or only an adjunct to individual therapy. The work often goes much deeper than imagined. Group therapy provides support for change; reductions in isolation, stigma, guilt, and shame; opportunities to rehearse new behaviors; feedback to support a more authentic self-image; a way to overcome denial through listening to others describe similar situations; sharing of coping skills; and confrontation without shame, because other group members have also "been there."

TABLE 11–3. Challenging relationship myths

Patient belief	Challenge statement
1. I can't stand it if my partner gets upset with me.	It may be temporarily uncomfortable if my partner is upset with me, but I will be okay.
2. I don't deserve to get what I want or need in a relationship.	My wants and needs are valid, and I deserve to get my wants and needs met in a relationship.
3. In a relationship, I should be willing to sacrifice my own needs for my partner.	It is essential to recognize and communicate my needs to my partner; sacrificing my needs does not foster a healthy relationship based on equality.
4. If this relationship comes to an end, it will destroy me.	I may experience painful emotions if the relationship ends, but I will ultimately be okay. I am not defined by this one relationship.
5. Saying no or setting limits with my partner is a selfish thing to do.	Setting limits and saying no are important ways to protect both myself and the relationship.

Source. Adapted from Linehan 1993.

Psychopharmacological Treatments

There are no accepted psychopharmacological interventions currently available for romantic relationship addiction. Psychotropic medication might be used to target specific symptoms for these patients—such as insomnia—as well as co-occurring disorders.

That said, recent research suggests that adjunctive drug-based therapies may help facilitate the treatment of romantic relationship addiction by working on neurochemical substrates. Three emotion-motivation subsystems have been identified that may be involved in destructive love patterns: lust, attraction, and attachment. Differential pharmacotherapies are proposed to target each area. Examples include the following: 1) oral naltrexone as an antilust treatment targeting craving; 2) obsessive-compulsive disorder medications as an anti-attraction treatment targeting obsessive romantic thinking; and 3) oxytocin/dopamine antagonists as an anti-attachment treatment (Earp et al. 2013).

Earp et al. (2013) outlined several conditions for the ethical use of "anti-love technologies." These conditions include 1) establishing that clear harm results from the addictive relationship; 2) confirming informed consent; 3) establishing that the treatment can decrease impulsiveness and help the person follow higher-order goals; and 4) noting that other, nonbiotechnological methods have failed and/or have been considered. Safety and efficacy of these potential treatments need to be established prior to their use.

Self-Help and Support Systems

There are tens of thousands of people who identify themselves as addicts of various types. In 12-step meetings across the country and online, they bring and share many decades of collective experience with the struggle, suffering, and recovery of their particular addiction. They are not therapy groups—although therapeutic effects are reported—and they are led by members, not therapists. A 12-step program is a fellowship in which participants share their experience, hope, and strength in order to help themselves and others. The 12 steps are a set of suggestions that enhance addicted individual's ability to remain abstinent "one day at a time" from their addictions. The steps have to do with acknowledging the many things we have no control over, acknowledging a power greater than ourselves, honesty, forgiveness, making amends for past transgressions, and service to others.

SLAA is a 12-step program specific to love and sex addictions. Forming meaningful connections with others in the context of recovery can diffuse the complete reliance on one central attachment figure, which is so prominent in romantic relationship addiction. These connections may also result in decreased feelings of dependency. When Jenny began to attend meetings (AA and

SLAA, at first, then AA only), she set goals for herself to spend time with females in recovery as opposed to looking for another relationship with a man. This is but one example of how the program can help.

Conclusion

There are myriad treatment approaches that can be used to effectively address romantic relationship addiction; the common thread among all techniques is a strong therapeutic relationship. Alliance has been repeatedly demonstrated to be the most robust predictor of treatment success in psychotherapy research (Safran and Muran 2000), and it is of particular import when treating clients whose presenting problem directly relates to interpersonal functioning in the context of close, intimate relationships.

Key Points

- Romantic relationship addiction is just like chemical and behavioral addictions in its psychological, chemical, and neuroanatomical aspects.

- Romantic relationship addiction is not an addiction to mature, healthy love. It is an obsessive and compulsive approach to the euphoria of attraction or the hope and promise of attachment. It typically becomes an addiction in those individuals who have had conflicted attachments or traumatic experiences in childhood.

- Recovery from this addiction can be seen in characteristics such as realistic expectations of relationships; balanced interest and investment in self and partner; development of an independent identity, with one's own set of interests, friends, and commitments; development of honesty and trust; and the establishment and maintenance of personal limits and boundaries.

References

American Psychiatric Association: Diagnostic and Statistical Manual of Mental Disorders, 5th Edition. Arlington, VA, American Psychiatric Association, 2013

The Augustine Fellowship, SLAA: Characteristics of Sex and Love Addiction. San Antonio, TX, Fellowship-Wide Services, 1990

Beattie M: Codependent No More: How to Stop Controlling Others and Care for Yourself, 2nd Revised Edition. Center City, MN, Hazelden Publishing, 1986

Bowlby J: A Secure Base. New York, Basic Books, 1988

Burkett JP, Young LJ: The behavioral, anatomical and pharmacological parallels between social attachment, love and addiction. Psychopharmacology (Berl) 224(1):1–26, 2012 22885871

Earp BD, Wudarczyk OA, Sandberg A, et al: If I could just stop loving you: anti-love biotechnology and the ethics of a chemical breakup. Am J Bioeth 13(11):3–17, 2013 24161170

Fisher HE, Brown LL, Aron A, et al: Reward, addiction, and emotion regulation systems associated with rejection in love. J Neurophysiol 104(1):51–60, 2010 20445032

Hartney E: What is love addiction? February 15, 2013. Available at http://addictions.about.com/od/LoveAddiction/a/What-Is-Love-Addiction.htm. Accessed February 8, 2014.

Holmes J: Attachment, Intimacy, Autonomy: Using Attachment Theory in Adult Psychotherapy. New York, Jason Aronson, 1996

Linehan M: Skills Training Manual for Borderline Personality Disorder. New York, Guilford, 1993

Miller W, Rollnick S: Motivational Interviewing, 2nd Edition. New York, Guilford, 2002

Moore JD: Confusing Love With Obsession: When Being in Love Means Being in Control. Center City, MN, Hazelden Publishing, 2010

Norwood R: Women Who Love Too Much. New York, Simon & Schuster, 1979

Potenza MN: The neurobiology of pathological gambling and drug addiction. Philos Trans R Soc Lond B Biol Sci 363(1507):3181–3189, 2008

Safran JD, Muran, JC: Negotiating the Therapeutic Alliance: A Relational Treatment Guide. New York, Guilford, 2000

Smith DE: The process addictions and the new ASAM definition of addiction. J Psychoactive Drugs 44(1):1–4, 2012 22641960

Questions

1.   Which of the following is NOT a characteristic of romantic relationship addiction?

   A. Withdrawal.
   B. Craving.
   C. Tolerance.
   D. Desire for intimacy.
   E. Functional impairment.

The correct answer is D.

Romantic relationship addiction shares many of the same criteria as substance use disorder in DSM-5, including withdrawal, craving, tolerance, and functional impairment. In romantic relationship addiction, withdrawal manifests as anxiety, panic, and grief when faced with episodes of separation or when the relationship ends; craving manifests as wanting to spend time with the partner above all else and often to the exclusion of most all other activities; tolerance manifests as escalating demands on the love interest; and functional impairment can manifest in a number of ways, such as remaining in emotionally, physically, or sexually abusive relationships; reducing time spent at work or with family and friends; and depressive symptoms induced by loss, separation, or fear of separation. In romantic relationship addiction, there is a fear of true intimacy, whereas desire for intimacy is a characteristic of normative, healthy attachment.

2.   Treatment for romantic relationship addiction may include

    A. Motivational interviewing.
    B. Dialectical behavior therapy.
    C. Cognitive-behavioral therapy.
    D. Self-help/support groups.
    E. All of the above.

The correct answer is E.

Treatment for romantic relationship addiction may include any and/or all of the above treatments, depending on the individual patient, the specific presenting issue, and the skill set of the treating therapist. Treatment should cater to the individual, and multiple techniques and modalities may be woven into the treatment in order to maximize potential benefit and give the patient multiple coping strategies.

3.   Which of the following is NOT a potential benefit of attending self-help/support groups such as Sex and Love Addicts Anonymous (SLAA)?

    A. Decreased isolation.
    B. Monitoring internal dialogue.
    C. Validation and normalization of patient's experience.
    D. Decreased feelings of shame.
    E. Decreased dependency on primary partner.

The correct answer is B.

Cognitive-behavioral therapy helps patients to identify distortions in thinking by, among other things, monitoring their internal dialogue. Self-help/support groups such as SLAA can help individuals to feel less alone and to feel the support of a community of people with similar issues. This may decrease feelings of shame and alienation and may help to increase autonomy as the individual becomes less dependent on the object of his or her compulsive attachment.

CHAPTER 12

Shopping Addiction

If the Shoe Fits,
Buy It in Every Color!

Najeeb Hussain, M.D.
Nicole Guanci, M.D.
Mahreen Raza, M.D.
Dmitry Ostrovsky, B.A.

SHOPPING is an extremely popular pastime in the United States. Studies estimate that Americans spend approximately 6 hours per week shopping (Grant et al. 2011). This common behavior becomes pathological when an individual cannot control the time and/or money dedicated to shopping. Negative consequences that ensue include accumulation of debt, feelings of guilt, and relational problems. In the literature, pathological shopping has historically been referred to as compulsive buying disorder. Although still poorly understood, there is a rising consensus that psychological and biological parallels exist between compulsive buying disorder and the substance use addictions. This has led to a more recent classification of pathological shopping as shopping addiction. The shift from a compulsive to an addictive nosology has been appreciated by psychiatrists, and a proposed revision for DSM-5 (American Psychiatric Association 2013) included adding shopping addiction to the category of addiction and related behaviors (O'Brien 2010).

Clinical Case

Sandra is a 35-year-old white woman who, for the past 3 years, has been treated for anxiety and depression with alprazolam, prescribed by her primary medical doctor (PMD). She was referred to the outpatient psychiatry clinic by her PMD for the evaluation of shopping sprees. Sandra reports worsening anxiety over the course of several months. She complains of relational problems with her husband, whom she describes as "never around." She expresses anxiety in handling the responsibility of raising her two young children, as well as feeling pressured at work by her boss. Sandra explains that her doctor is concerned about shopping sprees that she describes to him. She elaborates that she spends at least $1,000 per week on shoes and clothes. She notices that she shops more when she feels anxious and experiences a sense of relief when completing a purchase. She describes this as "feeling at peace for just a little bit." She admits that sometimes she buys items she cannot afford, has accumulated credit card debt close to $10,000, and has piles of unopened boxes of clothing in her garage. She also admits that her husband often yells at her for shopping excessively and for causing financial strain on the family. During the interview, she recalls that when she was growing up, she would "escape" with her mother and go shopping when her father was "in a mood." She also clarified that her shopping sprees do not occur exclusively when she is feeling depressed. Rather, she expresses guilt because of all of the time and money she devotes to shopping, stating, "I should be spending more time with my kids instead." She also describes some irritability, restlessness, and difficulty falling asleep. She denies any hypomanic, manic, psychotic, or obsessive-compulsive symptoms. She denies any changes in shopping behavior associated with her current medication. She denies any alcohol or illicit drug use.

Sandra began taking citalopram 10 mg/day for the treatment of anxiety symptoms. Biweekly cognitive-behavioral therapy (CBT) sessions are also recommended. Over the course of 3 months of pharmacotherapy, alprazolam was titrated and discontinued. Sandra reports improvement in her anxiety symptoms and decreased urges to shop. She reports improvement in sleep and "not flying off the handle as much" at her family. She notes that her relationship with her husband has improved since she "stopped racking up bills" because of her shopping. She also admits to doing better at work when she does not feel pressured to leave early to beat the traffic to the mall. Through her psychotherapy sessions, she is able to identify coping strategies to deal with her urges to shop. Instead of grabbing her credit card and heading for the nearest mall, she is learning how to identify other strategies for dealing with stress. She decides that having dinner with her husband and playing in the backyard with the children are better options. With the implementation of these strategies, Sandra is getting along better both at home and at work.

Discussion

Sandra described shopping behaviors that are considered consistent with a diagnosis of shopping addiction; however, this is not currently categorized in DSM-5. Her patterns of behavior related to shopping and the resultant ramifications on her social and work functioning also met criteria proposed by McElroy et al. (1994), which have been used in the literature to describe addictive shopping behavior. Sandra clearly described negative effects at work and at home, financial difficulties, negative feelings associated with her behaviors, and repetitive "urges" to shop. Similar to the pattern of emotion in substance addictions, Sandra experienced an impulse to shop in order to curb negative feelings, then a short-lived surge of positive feelings, followed by a resurgence of negative emotions, mainly guilt and shame.

Like many individuals with behavioral addictions, Sandra likely had a concomitant anxiety disorder. Because of her anxiety symptoms and some support from the literature (Karim and Chaudhri 2012) involving improved response with selective serotonin reuptake inhibitors, she began taking citalopram. CBT was also incorporated into therapy because studies (Aboujaoude et al. 2003; Mueller et al. 2011) also supported its use in treatment of shopping addiction.

With both psychotherapy and pharmacotherapy, Sandra reported symptom improvement in both anxiety and shopping behaviors. She was able to identify other coping mechanisms, which she incorporated into her daily life with little trouble. She reported less shopping and less debt as a result. She also experienced less tension at home and at work. She continued pharmacotherapy with citalopram, which was titrated to 20 mg/day. At the latest session, she also discussed joining a Shoppers Anonymous group at her local church, in order to share her story and learn from others with similar issues.

History

Recent media attention misleadingly implies that compulsive buying is a new phenomenon. However, compulsive buying was first described in the psychiatric literature in the early 1900s. Emil Kraepelin and Eugen Bleuler (Aboujaoude et al. 2003) both classified compulsive buying as one of the "impulsive insanities," along with kleptomania and pyromania (Karim and Chaudhri 2012). Originally termed *oniomania*, roughly translated as "buying mania," it is a concept that continues to be poorly understood and classified (Aboujaoude et al. 2003). It has proven difficult to differentiate between normal shopping behaviors, intermittent splurges, and compulsive shopping (Karim and Chaudhri 2012). In the 1990s and 2000s, there was an interest in classifying compulsive buying under the "obsessive compulsive spectrum" (Black 2001). However, according to the DSM-5 Task Force, compulsive buying is a poor match for obsessive-compulsive spectrum disorders because of its different phenomenology, lack of family history of obsessive-compulsive disorder, and different treatment response (Black 2001).

Etiology

The etiology of compulsive buying is poorly understood. Studies have implicated opiate, serotonergic, and dopaminergic systems (Karim and Chaudhri 2012). A key finding comes from studies on Parkinson's disease, in which patients prescribed L-dopa or dopamine agonists tended to have higher rates of compulsive buying (Karim and Chaudhri 2012). This suggests that dopamine may play a key role in compulsive shopping, similar to its role in drug addiction. This parallel to drug addiction is supported by the finding that the brain does not distinguish between dopamine release in the nucleus accumbens and ventral tegmental area secondary to drug use or experience (like shopping) (Hartston 2012). Furthermore, functional neuroimaging studies have shown that shopping activates many of the same brain regions as drugs of abuse, specifically the mesocorticolimbic system and the amygdala (Olsen 2011). Recent evidence suggests that behavioral addictions may lead to neuroadaptations similar to those reported with substance addictions, including a hijacking of the neural circuits responsible for the natural reward pathways. If a drug or experience is hyperstimulating, this neuroadaptation (namely, downregulation of dopamine receptors) occurs with repeated exposures.

For shopping, several factors may contribute to increased addictive potential. Neuromarketing has been used to create hyperstimulating experiences for shoppers, and online shopping has increased the exposure to shopping. Individuals are now able to shop at any time, in any location, and across a variety of genres with just a few clicks (Hartston 2012). In fact, Internet shopping has been estimated to account for 70% of all purchases (Kukar-Kinney et al. 2009). Kukar-Kinney et al. (2009) found that individuals with higher compulsive buying tendencies prefer shopping online because of the immediate positive feelings that may be evoked by "Express Checkout," in addition to the benefit of avoiding family/friends, retailers, and social interactions that may worsen underlying feelings of guilt and shame. Shopping addiction also has mood components. Studies have shown that compulsive shopping can help individuals relieve negative feelings by creating a temporary "high" similar to substance addiction. Thus it follows that alleviation of negative feelings by shopping provides reinforcement of the behavior. It also follows that Internet shopping provides a faster relief than traditional store shopping, which further potentiates the addictive potential when shopping behavior involves the Internet (Kukar-Kinney et al. 2009).

Other factors that influence compulsive shopping include buying motives. Kukar-Kinney et al. (2009) described hedonic motives, which refer to positive feelings associated with shopping, such as pleasure and excitement. Cultural and environmental factors may also contribute, particularly the number of hours spent watching television (Grant et al. 2011) and the degree of materialism within the individual's society or social group (Mueller et al. 2011).

Genetics

Studies investigating the behavioral genomics of compulsive shopping have found that patients with compulsive shopping have family histories of mood disorders, substance abuse, anxiety disorders, and compulsive buying disorders—a finding also consistent with the substance use disorders (Black 2001). Other studies attempting to elucidate the genetics of shopping addiction have not shown definitive findings. In one study, there were no associations found between two serotonin (*5-HTT*) transporter gene polymorphisms in people with and without compulsive shopping behavior (Black 2001). Studies identifying the role of serotonin in shopping addiction have shown mixed results.

Epidemiology

Epidemiological reports suggest a 2%–8% prevalence of compulsive shopping in the United States (Karim and Chaudhri 2012), with the latest reports estimating between 5.8% and 8.9% (see Table 12–1; Kukar-Kinney et al. 2009). The data on gender differences in compulsive buying disorder are mixed, mostly because of the greater preponderance of women included in studies (Karim and Chaudhri 2012). Estimates of a gender ratio of 9:1 (female to male) have been suggested, whereas others report ratios nearly equal (Karim and Chaudhri 2012). This disorder has been reported worldwide, but it appears to be overrepresented in developed countries and among the wealthy elite in underdeveloped countries. Age of onset is usually around 18–30 years old (Karim and Chaudhri 2012).

Studies suggest that most compulsive shopping begins during adolescence, when individuals acquire credit cards and become more financially independent. In a study by Grant et al. (2011), high school students were surveyed, and 3.5% were found to have a shopping problem. This was also associated with smoking, drug use, sadness/hopelessness, and antisocial behaviors. Furthermore, these students endorsed urges to buy, attempts to cut back on shopping, a calming effect from the act of making the purchase, and negative consequences due to shopping. These aspects make compulsive shopping appear similar to other substance addictions (Grant et al. 2011).

Assessment

The Compulsive Buying Scale is based on the criteria of McElroy et al. (1994). It defines compulsive buyers as individuals scoring at least 2 standard deviations less than the mean (on the questionnaire) and has been found to correctly classify 88% of individuals tested (Black 2001). Another scale, proposed by Valence et al. (1988), called the Compulsive Buying Measurement Scale, consists of 16 items in four dimensions (tendency to spend, feeling the urge to buy or shop, postpurchase guilt, and family environment) (Black 2001). Christenson et al. (1994) developed the Minnesota Impulsive Disorder Interview, which is used to assess the presence of compulsive buying, kleptomania, trichotilloma-

TABLE 12–1.   Prevalence rates for compulsive behaviors in the United States

Disorder	Rate
Pathological gambling	1%–2%
Compulsive sexual behavior	3%–6%
Binge-eating disorder	2%–3%
Compulsive buying	5.8%–8.9%

Source.   Data from Karim and Chaudhri 2012.

nia, intermittent explosive disorder, pathological gambling, compulsive sexual behavior, and compulsive exercise (Black 2001).

Diagnosis

A diagnosis of shopping addiction is not included in DSM-5. At this time, there is not enough evidence to establish diagnostic criteria for these "repetitive behaviors" to be classified as mental disorders (American Psychiatric Association 2013).

The literature defines *compulsive buying disorder* as a disorder associated with compulsive thoughts or impulses to purchase unnecessary or large amounts of items despite negative consequences. The disorder is associated with unpleasant tension and an urge to perform an enjoyable act even though it causes significant distress at a later time (Karim and Chaudhri 2012). To further delineate these behaviors, McElroy et al. (1994) have developed diagnostic criteria as defined in Table 12–2.

Black (2001) has reported that individuals with compulsive buying disorder are preoccupied with shopping and spending. The behavior typically consumes many hours per week. Four distinct phases of compulsive buying disorder have been described: anticipation, preparation, shopping, and spending (Karim and Chaudhri 2012). It has been reported that negative emotions, such as anger, anxiety, boredom, and self-critical thought, were the most common antecedents to shopping binges, whereas euphoria or relief of negative emotions were the most common immediate consequences (Karim and Chaudhri 2012).

In addition to biological similarities, compulsive buying disorder shares distinct psychological and behavioral features with substance addiction. These include the following: preoccupation with the activity, spending significant amounts of time and money on the activity, a high degree of ritualization about the activity, relief of negative emotions associated with the activity, range in frequency dependent on personal funds, and resultant feelings of guilt and shame

---

TABLE 12–2.   Criteria for compulsive buying disorder

1. Frequent preoccupation with shopping or intrusive, irresistible, "senseless" buying impulses
2. Clearly buying more than needed or can be afforded
3. Distress related to buying behavior
4. Significant interference with work or social functioning

Source.   Adapted from McElroy et al. 1994.

(Karim and Chaudhri 2012). Christenson et al. (1994) and Schlosser et al. (1994) found that pathological shopping behaviors are not typically confined to special holidays or birthdays (Black 2001). The study also found that most pathological shoppers prefer to shop alone, describe experiences enhanced by sensory experiences of product placement (and being in the actual store), and leave unopened, stacked boxes of unnecessary items around the house (Black 2001).

Comorbid Disorders

Compulsive buying disorder is often comorbid with mood disorders (21%–100%), eating disorders (8%–85%), substance use disorders (24%–46%), other impulse-control disorders, and personality disorders (60%) (see Table 12–3) (Karim and Chaudhri 2012). In studies of depressed patients, compulsive shopping was associated with a high level of impulsivity and novelty seeking in addition to higher rates of recurrent depressive episodes, bipolar disorder, bulimia, kleptomania, benzodiazepine abuse, and suicide attempts (Black 2001). Schlosser et al. (1994) found that at least 60% of compulsive buyers met criteria for personality disorders, including obsessive-compulsive personality disorder (22%), borderline personality disorder (15%), and avoidant personality disorder (15%) (Black 2001).

Treatments

Pharmacotherapy

There is emerging evidence that pharmacotherapies used in treating drug addiction may be promising options for nondrug addictions. For example, naltrexone (Kim et al. 2001), nalmefene, *N*-acetylcysteine, and modafinil have all been reported to reduce craving in pathological gamblers (Leung and Cottler 2009).

There is no standard pharmacological treatment for shopping addiction at this time. Some clinical studies suggest that citalopram may have some beneficial effects in preventing relapse in compulsive-buying disorder patients (Karim and

TABLE 12–3.   Comorbidities associated with shopping addiction

Mood disorders	21%–100%
Anxiety disorders	40%
Substance use disorders	24%–46%
Eating disorders	8%–85%
Impulse control disorders	35%
Personality disorders	60%

Source.   Data from Karim and Chaudhri 2012; McElroy et al. 1994.

Chaudhri 2012). However, the use of other selective serotonin reuptake inhibitors, such as fluvoxamine, has shown mixed results. In one double-blind, placebo-controlled trial, citalopram resulted in a 63% response rate (Aboujaoude et al. 2003). In two double-blind trials, fluvoxamine failed to show an improvement in response rate over the placebo (Aboujaoude et al. 2003). In an open-label study by Aboujaoude et al. (2003), 24 subjects meeting diagnostic criteria suggested by McElroy et al. (1994) were enrolled in a 12-week open-label trial of citalopram; dosages ranged from 20 mg/day to 60 mg/day. This study found a 71% response rate as measured by the Clinical Global Impression–Improvement Scale and the Yale-Brown Obsessive Compulsive Scale–Shopping Version (Aboujaoude et al. 2003). A 12-month follow-up of responders showed that the majority remained in remission at 12 months (Aboujaoude et al. 2003). However, no clear association was demonstrated between remission status during follow-up and continued use of citalopram at the therapeutic dose established in the open-label trial. However, a subsequent 9-week double-blind, placebo-controlled study showed a 63% relapse rate on placebo treatment versus a 0% relapse rate on continued citalopram treatment (Aboujaoude et al. 2003). Response to citalopram was associated with a higher likelihood of remission over the course of 1 year. Other studies have suggested that mood stabilizers may be potentially useful (Black 2001).

Psychotherapy

Studies suggest that CBT, dialectical behavioral therapy, and psychodynamic psychotherapy may have promising results in treating compulsive buying disorder (Müller et al. 2013). CBT focuses on factors that maintain and reinforce the problematic buying behavior and delineates strategies for controlling impulsive spending. Maintaining a diary to identify triggers, describe the shopping behavior itself, and record the consequences of compulsive shopping assists patients in understanding behaviors from a different perspective. Additional options include 12-step programs, such as Debtors Anonymous, debt consolidation, and credit counseling (see Table 12–4) (Black 2001).

TABLE 12–4.	Shopping hygiene tips

1. Use cash or debit cards when shopping.

2. Lower open credit on each card account to the minimum value.

3. Ask a family member or a friend to accompany when shopping.

4. Adopt healthy alternatives, such as yoga, acupuncture, exercise, walking, or window-shopping, to reduce stress.

5. Seek help for debt consolidation and credit counseling.

6. Use resources such as Debtors Anonymous.

7. Minimize exposure to advertisements in, for example, electronic media and print media.

Source. Data from Black 2001.

Key Points

- Shopping addiction is not classified as a mental disorder in DSM-5.

- People who are addicted to shopping exhibit significant behavioral and biological similarities to people who with substance addictions.

- Dopamine likely plays a key role in shopping addiction.

- Shopping addiction is more common in women in developed countries.

- Epidemiological reports suggest a 2%–8% prevalence of compulsive shopping in the United States.

- Mood disorders, substance use disorders, and personality disorders are often comorbid with shopping addiction.

- There is no standard pharmacological treatment for shopping addiction at this time; however, some studies support the use of selective serotonin reuptake inhibitors and cognitive-behavioral therapy.

References

Aboujaoude E, Gamel N, Koran LM: A 1-year naturalistic follow-up of patients with compulsive shopping disorder. J Clin Psychiatry 64(8):946–950, 2003 12927011

American Psychiatric Association: Diagnostic and Statistical Manual of Mental Disorders, 5th Edition. Arlington, VA, American Psychiatric Association, 2013

Black DW: Compulsive buying disorder: definition, assessment, epidemiology and clinical management. CNS Drugs 15(1):17–27, 2001 11465011

Christenson GA, Faber RJ, deZwaan M, Raymond NC, et al: Compulsive buying: descriptive characteristics and psychiatric comorbidity. J Clin Psychiatry 55(1):5–11, 1994 8294395

Grant JE, Potenza MN, Krishnan-Sarin S, et al: Shopping problems among high school students. Compr Psychiatry 52(3):247–252, 2011 21497217

Hartston H: The case for compulsive shopping as an addiction. J Psychoactive Drugs 44(1):64–67, 2012 22641966

Karim R, Chaudhri P: Behavioral addictions: an overview. J Psychoactive Drugs 44(1):5–17, 2012 22641961

Kim SW, Grant JE, Adson DE, et al: Double-blind naltrexone and placebo comparison study in the treatment of pathological gambling. Biol Psychiatry 49(11):914–921, 2001 11377409

Kukar-Kinney M, Ridgway NM, Monroe KB: The relationship between consumers' tendencies to buy compulsively and their motivations to shop and buy on the Internet. Journal of Retailing 85(3):298–307, 2009

Leung KS, Cottler LB: Treatment of pathological gambling. Curr Opin Psychiatry 22(1):69–74, 2009 19122538

McElroy S, Keck PE Jr, Pope HG Jr, Smith JM, et al: Compulsive buying: a report of 20 cases. J Clin Psychiatry 55(6):242–248, 1994 8071278

Mueller A, Mitchell JE, Peterson LA, et al: Depression, materialism, and excessive Internet use in relation to compulsive buying. Compr Psychiatry 52(4):420–424, 2011 21683178

Müller A, Arikian A, de Zwaan M, et al: Cognitive-behavioural group therapy versus guided self-help for compulsive buying disorder: a preliminary study. Clin Psychol Psychother 20(1):28–35, 2013 21823199

O'Brien CP: Commentary on Tao et al. (2010): Internet addiction and DSM-V. Addiction 105:565, 2010

Olsen CM: Natural rewards, neuroplasticity, and non-drug addictions. Neuropharmacology 61(7):1109–1122, 2011 21459101

Schlosser S, Black DW, Repertinger S, Freet D: Compulsive buying. demography, phenomenology, and comorbidity in 46 subjects. Gen Hosp Psychiatry 16(3):205–212, 1994 8063088

Tao R, Huang X, Wang J, et al: Proposed diagnostic criteria for Internet addiction. Addiction 105(3):556–564, 2010 20403001

Valence G, D'Astous A, Fortier L: Compulsive buying: concept and measurement. J Consum Policy 11(4):419–433, 1988

Questions

1. Which of the following emotions most likely occurs prior to a shopping binge?

    A. Anger.

    B. Anxiety.

    C. Boredom.

    D. All of the above.

The correct answer is D.

It has been reported that negative emotions, such as anger, anxiety, and boredom, and self-critical thought are the most common antecedents to shopping binges. Euphoria or relief of negative emotions is the most common immediate consequence. These emotions highly resemble the negative feelings—and subsequent relief of negative feelings—typically associated with substance addictions.

2. Which class of medications is NOT a potential treatment for shopping addiction?

    A. Selective serotonin reuptake inhibitors.
    B. Benzodiazepines.
    C. Opioid antagonists.
    D. Mood stabilizers.

The correct answer is B.

Studies have shown that selective serotonin reuptake inhibitors, particularly citalopram, have a potential benefit for patients with shopping addiction. Other studies have suggested the potential use of opioid antagonists (including naltrexone) and mood stabilizers. Benzodiazepines have not been used to treat shopping addiction.

3. A 24-year-old woman presents with engaging in shopping sprees, which occur during times of stress. This shopping behavior has resulted in significant debt and has begun to interfere with her job and relationships. She is often distressed after these sprees yet cannot resist the impulse to buy. Which of the following, if true, makes shopping addiction a more likely diagnosis than bipolar disorder?

    A. Preoccupation with shopping and impulses to buy.
    B. Periods of decreased need for sleep accompanying buying episodes.
    C. Psychotic symptoms accompanying buying episodes.
    D. Interference in work or social functioning.

The correct answer is A.

The criteria proposed for shopping addiction include frequent preoccupation with shopping or intrusive, irresistible buying impulses; clearly buying more than needed or afforded; distress related to buying behavior; and significant interference with work or social functioning. Option

D is similar to both shopping addiction and bipolar disorder. Option B would make bipolar disorder more likely. Option C is not a criterion for either shopping addiction or bipolar disorder.

CHAPTER 13

Tanning Addiction

When Orange Is the New Bronze

Petros Levounis, M.D., M.A.
Omar Mohamed, B.A.
Carolyn J. Heckman, Ph.D.

"**WHITE** skin makes up for seven defects" says an eighth century Japanese proverb (Wagatsuma 1968, p. 129), and for a long time, pale skin was the standard of beauty in both Eastern and Western cultures. All that changed in the early years of the twentieth century when tanning started becoming first accepted and then highly sought after, leading to Coco Chanel's famous quote: "The 1929 girl must be tanned. A golden tan is the index of chic!" (cited by Randle 1997, p. 462). Almost overnight, the light switch was turned on, and darkly tanned skin became the indisputable benchmark of good looks.

Nowadays, while most people are well aware of the dangers of tanning, both from the sun and from indoor tanning sun beds, they are also ambivalent—if not torn—by society's mixed messages. On one hand, science unequivocally has linked ultraviolet (UV) light exposure with cancer, but, on the other hand, the social pressure to conform to the tanned ideal is alive and well in the twenty-first century. The distribution of people along the axis of tanning intensity, from no tanning to extreme exposure, may resemble a Gaussian curve. On the left, some people have eliminated tanning completely from their lives; in the middle, the majority have adopted a cautious moderation approach using sunscreen and avoiding prolonged exposures; and, on the right, at the other end of the spectrum, we find a small number of people who tan excessively and most likely pathologically. The risk factors, biopsychosocial-spiritual determinants, co-

187

morbid illnesses, clinical presentation, and course of illness of this third group of people seem to resemble moderate to severe substance use disorders and other behavioral addictions such as gambling and Internet gaming (Levounis and Herron 2014).

Clinical Case

Giselle is an attractive, talented, and motivated 22-year-old woman from New Jersey who fills the room with her exuberance and charm. A valedictorian at her high school, she now attends Columbia University, double majors in political science and English, and is on track to go to law school at practically any school she chooses. Young and brilliant, she is determined to one day become an unassailable civil rights prosecutor. Even though she has a "work hard, play later mentality," she always finds time to let loose and party with friends.

Giselle and her two older sisters were raised in a loving Irish Italian family, but they lost their mother to breast cancer when Giselle was only 6 years old. Having been brought up by a single father, Giselle is more independent and mature than most of her friends. Her boyfriend Nick, whom she met right out of high school, is just as driven and successful. He is a second-year medical student at New York University, with an eye to becoming an orthopedic surgeon. Their relationship has been nothing short of perfect, as though it had been pulled out of a fairy tale written by the Brothers Grimm. Giselle has been climbing the ladder of success, and it seems like nothing can get in her way.

Giselle was first exposed to suntanning at a very young age. Growing up at the New Jersey shore, she would go to the beach with her father and sisters frequently. While Giselle played in the sand, she would watch her siblings lie on the beach and tan. She constantly overheard them talk about how they loved being tan and how beautiful it made them look. Wanting to be tan and beautiful just like her sisters, she ditched the sand and began tanning right next to them. Giselle continued to tan every summer throughout her preteen and teen years, right through middle school and into high school.

When Giselle started high school, a new a popular television show was launched on MTV called *Jersey Shore*. Because she was from that area, Giselle loved watching the series, and Snooki quickly became her favorite. The stars of the show were praised for their tanned skin and were frequently filmed tanning on the beach or in a salon. Indoor tanning was a new trend, and Giselle was already ahead of all of her friends. Conveniently, a new tanning salon opened in her town, and what used to be an activity she participated in only during the summer months now became a year-round obligation. Frequency was limited at first, but it slowly started to increase. By the time she graduated from high school, Giselle was catching sun rays and UV light from tanning beds 5–6 times every month, year-round. She loved the way her skin looked and how tanning made her feel. Compliments flew in from every direction, even from her siblings and boyfriend. Tanning had such a positive effect on her life, and she saw no reason to stop.

College started, and freshman year turned out to be academically and socially more intense than she had expected. Giselle was always a great student, but she was having trouble acclimating to the demands of a college schedule—that was something she had never experienced before. She noticed that she always felt relaxed and stress-free after some UV rays. She began using tanning as a way to cope with stress. She bought an unlimited yearlong membership at her local tanning salon, and every morning she starts her day with a long relaxing tanning session. It is like her morning cup of coffee: she has to have it, her day simply cannot start without it. After every session, Giselle is relaxed and ready to face the world. By the end of her hectic day, all she can think about is the next session with her beloved UV rays.

Nick is the first to notice something different about Giselle's tanning habits. Because he is a medical student, he knows some of the dangers associated with chronic tanning. He notices the negative effects the chronic UV rays are having on her body. Her skin has begun to have a leathery texture and is covered in fine freckles (Lim et al. 2011). The young 22-year-old college student suddenly looks like a middle-aged mother. Nick loves his girlfriend very much and knows that he has to talk to her about her tanning. To him, Giselle is addicted to the UV rays. "Addicts use drugs; I'm too smart to be an addict," she said to Nick when he broached the subject.

Discussion

Tanning disorder is not currently listed as diagnosis in DSM-5 (American Psychiatric Association 2013). However, the Structured Interview for Tanning Abuse and Dependence (SITAD; Hillhouse et al. 2012) is a diagnostic tool based on DSM-IV-TR (American Psychiatric Association 2000) criteria for opioid use disorders. In order to meet tanning dependence criteria on the SITAD, Giselle would need to report three or more of the seven standard substance dependence symptoms with respect to tanning (e.g., tolerance to tanning, tanning withdrawal symptoms). If Giselle does not meet tanning dependence criteria on the SITAD, she would meet tanning abuse criteria if she continued recurrent tanning despite problems in a major life domain (i.e., work, school, home or safety, legal, social, and interpersonal arenas). There are also other measures of tanning pathology and dependence in the literature, some based on standard substance use measures, that could further assist in screening patients.

Given the case description, which included Giselle's daily tanning throughout the year, it is likely that she has experienced tolerance to tanning and withdrawal symptoms or has tanned to avoid withdrawal symptoms. It is unknown whether she would admit to additional diagnostic criteria, but she has probably been tanning longer or more frequently than intended and spends a great deal of time in tanning-related activities. Although it was not mentioned, she may have had a persistent desire or made unsuccessful attempts to cut down or control her tanning, or she has continued tanning despite knowledge of a persistent physical or psychological problem that is likely to have been caused or exacerbated by tanning. Thus Giselle would probably meet criteria for tanning use disorder, sometimes also referred to as tanning addiction. Alternative formulations of

Giselle's condition could classify her frequent tanning as a disorder of body image, anxiety, mood, or impulse control given the association of frequent tanning with such problems in the literature.

Giselle is similar to many other indoor tanners or people with symptoms of tanning addiction in that she began tanning during childhood or adolescence and is a young, white woman with older female family members who have served as tanning role models. Evidence has been mixed in terms of the association between indoor tanning and educational and socioeconomic status. In 2014, the Division of Cancer Prevention and Control of the Centers for Disease Control and Prevention released a major study of more than 25,000 high school students who answered the indoor tanning question on the 2009 and the 2011 national Youth Risk Behavior Survey (Guy et al. 2014). Indoor tanning (one or more times in the last year) was found to be highest among female, non-Hispanic white, and older high school students, and it was significantly associated with a cluster of potentially risky behaviors (see Table 13–1).

Giselle has been influenced by the television show *Jersey Shore* and, like others in her situation, has probably been exposed to a great deal of media, marketing, and misinformation portraying tanning as appealing, healthy, and safe. New York City, where Giselle attends college, also has a high density of tanning salons per square mile. Presumably, as valedictorian of her high school, attendance at an Ivy League university, and planning to attend law school, Giselle faces high levels of academic and achievement-oriented stress, which she admittedly addresses via her daily morning tanning sessions.

Treatments

Talking With Patients About Tanning

One intervention approach that has shown some promise in decreasing tanning and that is empirically supported for the treatment of substance use disorders is motivational interviewing (MI; Levounis and Arnaout 2010; Miller and Rollnick 2002). *MI* is a person-centered, guiding method of counseling used to elicit and strengthen motivation for change. The approach guides the individual to explore and attempt to resolve normal ambivalence about changing while increasing ambivalence or perceived discrepancy between current behavior and overall values. Self-motivational statements, or "change talk," are hypothesized to contribute greatly to changes in actual behavior. MI can be used as a treatment itself or to motivate individuals to engage in another form of treatment. One of the most difficult aspects of addiction treatment is engaging the patient in treatment. This may be especially true for a behavioral addiction such as tanning, which may not be taken seriously by some until the consequences are in-

TABLE 13–1. Behaviors associated with indoor tanning among high school students

Female and male students	Female students	Male students
Engaging in binge drinking	Using illegal drugs	Taking steroids without a physician's prescription
Using unhealthy weight control practices	Engaging in sexual intercourse with four or more persons in one's lifetime	Smoking cigarettes daily
Engaging in sexual intercourse		Attempting suicide

Source. Adapted from Guy et al. 2014.

disputable, such as developing a fatal melanoma. Here we discuss an approach to engage Giselle in treatment that is consistent with an MI or person-centered framework.

As with many individuals with mental or substance use disorders, Giselle may not be aware or willing to admit that she has a problem, particularly because tanning addiction is a relatively new construct. Thus one should approach the patient carefully, gauging her readiness to address the problem and enhancing the personal salience of the discussion along the way. It is generally helpful to initially focus on the reasons the patient has come for help and the problems that are bothering her rather than the patient's problems as perceived by the provider. However, Giselle does not seem to have experienced many negative consequences from tanning yet. Given the case description, what would most likely bring her into treatment would be pressure from or conflicts with her boyfriend regarding her excessive tanning. Nick seems to be more aware than Giselle about the problematic nature of her tanning behavior and its potential consequences. Because the relationship seems to be quite good and an important part of Giselle's life, the desire to maintain her romantic relationship would likely be highly motivating. Other possible motivators could be 1) a family member or close friend's diagnosis of malignant melanoma or 2) comorbid problems such as a body dysmorphic, eating, anxiety, or depressive disorder that she is no longer able to manage via tanning—despite the fact that her coping skills are probably fairly sophisticated given her academic and social success.

As Giselle begins to acknowledge the negative consequences of her tanning on her romantic relationship and other aspects of her life, it can be helpful to emphasize the connection between tanning and her perceived problems. Once rapport has been established and the patient has started to "open up," Giselle may become more interested in a description of the symptoms of tanning addiction and education about the effects of tanning on health and appearance. At that point in the patient's transition from the precontemplation to the contemplation stage of change (see discussion of the transtheoretical model given by Prochaska and DiClimente 1982), the clinician is typically tempted to launch into a heavily psychoeducational discourse and to provide a comprehensive list of the negative consequences of tanning. Instead, the clinician should continue to focus on what is most relevant to the patient. For example, appearance anxieties such as premature aging may be much more salient to a young woman such as Giselle compared with graver health concerns such as cancer. Even bright and high-functioning patients such as Giselle, who may think they are well informed about tanning, probably filter their view of the world through the distorted lens of their addiction.

Throughout Giselle's treatment, it is helpful to attempt to determine what is driving, reinforcing, and maintaining the tanning behavior. Giselle has received compliments on her appearance and feels more relaxed and less stressed after tanning. Thus Giselle would need to find other ways to feel attractive, receive compliments, manage stress, and relax. Does Giselle already use UV-free tanners and exercise regularly, or are there barriers to these healthier behaviors? UV-free tanning is safe as long as the chemicals are not inhaled. What other coping skills does Giselle possess, how successfully does she use them, and how can they be enhanced? For example, relaxation exercises, meditation, or yoga could be powerful stress relievers. If Giselle is unwilling to abstain from tanning, a harm-reduction approach could be used in an attempt to encourage Giselle to reduce the frequency, length, or intensity of her tanning sessions—or even to use sunscreen—to reduce the damage to her skin.

Psychosocial Treatments

Currently, treatment recommendations for excessive tanning are tentative suggestions built on successful treatments for other substance use disorders rather than being based on significant clinical experience or empirical evidence with tanners. Two approaches that have received preliminary empirical support in research (but not clinical) settings are MI and appearance-based interventions (Gibbons et al. 2005; Hillhouse and Turrisi 2002; Turrisi et al. 2008). These interventions have been shown to reduce indoor tanning but have not necessarily been shown to treat tanning addiction. One appearance-based intervention uses a special camera and software to create photos of UV radiation damage to the face in the form of freckles, dark spots, and wrinkles. Visually illustrating the appearance-related damage that has already been done may motivate patients to reduce their tanning behavior. In addition to MI, another treatment for substance use disorders that could potentially be applied to the treatment of tanning dependence is cognitive behavior therapy (CBT; Beck et al. 1979). In CBT, the clinician assists the patient in 1) modifying his or her dysfunctional thoughts about himself or herself, tanning, and his or her environment (e.g., "I look ugly when I'm pale") and 2) replacing his or her tanning behavior with healthier reinforcing alternatives, such as exercise. Interventions for similar or sometimes comorbid disorders that could potentially be applied to the treatment of tanning addiction include treatments for body dysmorphic, eating, depressive (with or without a seasonal pattern), and anxiety disorders. These treatments include psychosocial interventions such as CBT, as well as couples and family therapy. Although group therapy could potentially be quite helpful for excessive tanners (as it has been shown to be for substance use and other psychiatric disorders), it might be difficult to motivate patients to attend group sessions given the current lack of awareness, formal diagnosis, and treatment recommendations.

Pharmacological Treatments

At this point, the psychopharmacology of tanning addiction is limited to the treatment of potential comorbid disorders, primarily with antidepressants. Additionally, one study demonstrated that an opioid antagonist, naltrexone, induced withdrawal symptoms in frequent indoor tanners (Kaur et al. 2006). According to this line of research, it might be possible to extinguish tanning behavior if an addicted tanner were willing to take naltrexone consistently. If a patient in recovery were to slip and engage in tanning while taking naltrexone, he or she would not experience the usual reinforcing effects (i.e., relaxation and mood enhancement) of tanning and therefore would become less likely to relapse into the full addiction. More research is needed on this approach before it can be recommended for clinical use.

Community Resources

At this point, community resources for treatment of substance use and other psychiatric disorders may also be helpful for the treatment of tanning addiction. A team treatment approach that may include a counselor, psychiatrist, psychologist, dermatologist, primary care provider, and pediatrician, if appropriate, may be particularly helpful—especially if the patient suffers from comorbid disorders. Because tanning is most popular among children, adolescents, and young adults, it may be beneficial or required to involve the parents of the patient. Some treatment centers for substance use disorders are already advertising their services to tanners, but it is unclear on what clinical experience or empirical evidence such marketing is based.

With respect to prevention, some states have passed, or are currently in the process of passing, legislation to ban minors from indoor tanning because of its known association with skin cancer. Unfortunately, it has been shown that existing indoor tanning regulations pertaining to advertising, dosing, and mandatory warning labels are infrequently followed and enforced.

Key Points

- Viewing tanned skin as fashionable and attractive is a relatively recent phenomenon in U.S. history.

- Tanning disorder is not currently listed as official diagnosis in DSM-5.

- Opioid use disorder criteria have been applied to tanning behavior.

- Tanning and tanning addiction are most common in young, white women.

- Two approaches that have received preliminary empirical support for reducing engagement in tanning behavior in research (but not clinical) settings are motivational interviewing and appearance-based interventions.

- Ultraviolet-free tanning is safe as long as the chemicals are not inhaled.

- Naltrexone was shown to induce withdrawal symptoms in a small sample of frequent tanners.

- Currently, only a few states have banned minors from indoor tanning despite its known association with skin cancer and its potential for addiction.

References

American Psychiatric Association: Diagnostic and Statistical Manual of Mental Disorders, 4th Edition, Text Revision. Washington, DC, American Psychiatric Association, 2000

American Psychiatric Association: Diagnostic and Statistical Manual of Mental Disorders, 5th Edition. Arlington, VA, American Psychiatric Association, 2013

Beck A, Rush AJ, Shaw BF, et al: Cognitive Therapy of Depression. New York, Guilford, 1979

Gibbons FX, Gerrard M, Lane DJ, et al: Using UV photography to reduce use of tanning booths: a test of cognitive mediation. Health Psychol 24(4):358–363, 2005 16045371

Guy GP Jr, Berkowitz Z, Tai E, et al: Indoor tanning among high school students in the United States, 2009 and 2011. JAMA Dermatol 150(5):501–511, 2014 24577222

Hillhouse JJ, Turrisi R: Examination of the efficacy of an appearance-focused intervention to reduce UV exposure. J Behav Med 25(4):395–409, 2002 12136499

Hillhouse JJ, Baker MK, Turrisi R, et al: Evaluating a measure of tanning abuse and dependence. Arch Dermatol 148(7):815–819, 2012 22801615

Hunt Y, Augustson E, Rutten L, et al: History and culture of tanning in the United States, in Shedding Light on Indoor Tanning. Edited by Heckman CJ, Manne SL. New York, Springer, 2012, pp 5–31

Kaur M, Liguori A, Lang W, et al: Induction of withdrawal-like symptoms in a small randomized, controlled trial of opioid blockade in frequent tanners. J Am Acad Dermatol 54(4):709–711, 2006 16546596

Levounis P, Arnaout B (eds): Handbook of Motivation and Change: A Practical Guide for Clinicians. Washington, DC, American Psychiatric Publishing, 2010

Levounis P, Herron AJ (eds): The Addiction Casebook. Washington, DC, American Psychiatric Publishing, 2014

Lim HW, James WD, Rigel DS, et al: Adverse effects of ultraviolet radiation from the use of indoor tanning equipment: time to ban the tan. J Am Acad Dermatol 64(4):e51–e60, 2011 21295374

Miller WR, Rollnick S: Motivational Interviewing: Preparing People for Change, 2nd Edition. New York, Guilford, 2002

Prochaska JO, DiClemente CC: Transtheoretical therapy: toward a more integrative model of change. Psychotherapy 19:276–288, 1982

Randle HW: Suntanning: differences in perceptions throughout history. Mayo Clin Proc 72(5):461–466 1997 9146690

Turrisi R, Mastroleo NR, Stapleton J, et al: A comparison of 2 brief intervention approaches to reduce indoor tanning behavior in young women who indoor tan very frequently. Arch Dermatol 144(11):1521–1524, 2008 19015434

Wagatsuma H: The social perception of skin color in Japan, in Color and Race. Edited by Franklin JH. Boston, MA, Houghton Mifflin, 1968, pp 129–165

Questions

1. Which one of the following characteristics has been shown to be most likely associated with frequent indoor tanning?

   A. Higher socioeconomic status.
   B. Lower educational level.
   C. Presence of younger male siblings who are averse to tanning.
   D. Presence of older women in the family who have served as tanning role models.

   The correct answer is D.

   Frequent indoor tanners tend to be young, white women, who start going to tanning salons early in life and often model their behavior after older female family members with tanning behaviors. The evidence on any potential association between tanning behaviors and socioeconomic status or educational level has been equivocal. No studies have investigated younger brothers who are averse to tanning.

2. A patient with tanning addiction says, "I work hard and deserve a good tanning session at the end of a tough day at the office." Which one of the following responses is most consistent with the motivational interviewing approach?

   A. "No, you don't. Tanning will kill you and you know it."
   B. "I'm curious about the work ethic in your family, back when you were a kid."
   C. "It sounds like tanning has been one way for you to reward yourself."
   D. "I would like you to keep a daily record of the thoughts and feelings that you have around the time you leave work."

The correct answer is C.

Option C is an example of reflective listening, which along with open-ended questions, affirmations, reflections, and summaries forms the core strategies (the OARS) of motivational interviewing. Option A is a highly confrontational and provocative response that is rarely viewed to be constructive in twenty-first century psychotherapy. Option B is consistent with a psychodynamic approach, which aims to explore motives and underlying forces that determine human behavior. The homework exercise of option D, called "functional analysis," aims to determine the association between triggers (end of day) and responses (tanning session) in terms of automatic thoughts and feelings in preparation for "cognitive restructuring" and "coping skill building," all of which are elements of cognitive-behavior therapy.

3.   Which one of the following medications has shown some potential in the treatment of tanning addiction?

A. Naltrexone.
B. Dislufiram.
C. Varenicline.
D. Nalmefene.

The correct answer is A.

Naltrexone is a μ opioid receptor antagonist that has been studied for the treatment of many substance- and non-substance-related addictions, including alcohol, opioids, gambling, and tanning. In one small study, people who used indoor tanning heavily showed withdrawal symptoms in response to naltrexone, a finding that may have promising treatment implications. Nalmefene is also a μ opioid antagonist that has been investigated for the treatment of addiction to alcohol, gambling, and shopping but not tanning. Disulfiram blocks acetaldehyde dehydrogenase irreversibly and is used in the treatment of alcoholism, whereas varenicline is a partial agonist to the nicotinic acetylcholine receptor that successfully treats tobacco addiction.

CHAPTER 14

Work Addiction

Taking Care of Business

Michael S. Ascher, M.D.
Jonathan Avery, M.D.
Yael Holoshitz, M.D.

WORKAHOLISM as an addictive disorder is a relatively new concept in psychiatry. Unlike other addictions, excessive work is often viewed as an asset, and many cultures value those who prioritize work. A rewarding work life can be personally enriching, not to mention a necessary source of financial security. However, growing evidence suggests that a significant number of people struggle with excessive, compulsive, and detrimental work patterns. In a recent review article, Sussman (2012) noted that workaholism has a prevalence of 8%–17.5% among college educated people, possibly as high as 25% in certain populations, such as female attorneys, physicians, and mental health providers.

Wayne Oates first coined the term "workaholism" more than 40 years ago (Oates 1971). Since then it has become common parlance, with several different definitions. In clinical literature, the concept has been portrayed by hyperperformers, unhappy and obsessive individuals with low career success, or emotionally avoidant people more concerned with work than any other aspect of their lives (Griffiths 2011). Most definitions agree that a *workaholic* is someone who works excessively hard (behavioral component) and compulsively (cognitive component). *Workaholism* is a behavioral act with negative consequences, and an impulse beyond an individual's control. It may involve excessive time spent at work, difficulty disengaging from work, frustration and agitation when prevented from working, compulsive or inflexible working style, and negative life outcomes, including low self-esteem, high perceived stress, low life satisfaction, and poor performance. Ultimately, it may lead to burnout and ill health (Sussman 2012).

Workaholism is a true behavioral addiction and has features of the six core components of addiction (Griffiths and Karanika-Murray 2012). *Salience* occurs when work becomes the single most important activity in the person's life. This may dominate the person's thinking and preclude him or her from engaging in other meaningful activities because he or she is frequently preoccupied with work. *Mood modification* occurs when an individual uses work to either enhance his or her mood or to "numb" intolerable affects. *Tolerance* occurs when the amount of hours devoted to work steadily increases; often one may "chase the buzz" and attempt to replicate the initial pleasure experienced in intense work immersion. Withdrawal symptoms may be experienced as irritability, dysphoria, or moodiness when one is forced to disengage from work. *Conflict* may be experienced when the individual is forced to address other demands on his or her time, such as family. Conflict may be internal as insight is gained and a workaholic individual begins to realize that this compulsive behavior is causing undue distress. Finally, *relapse* describes the tendency for repeated return to unhealthy and compulsive patterns of work behavior.

Studies have shown that children of workaholic individuals are more likely to become workaholics themselves (Sussman 2012), and there is an association between an individual's own workaholism and that perceived of his or her parents. Disposition to workaholism includes achievement orientation and desire for higher self-esteem, stressful childhood, competition at work, and feeling more self-efficacious at work than in other settings. Frequently seen personality traits include obsessive compulsion, achievement orientation, perfectionism, and conscientiousness. Additionally, the tendency for overcontrol of the self and others may play a role in the etiology of workaholism, with more overcontrolling behavior associated with job involvement, stress, and work/nonwork conflict (Sussman 2012).

Workaholic individuals typically have a calamitous effect on themselves and their families. Research has shown that workaholics are at risk for sleep problems, weight gain, hypertension, anxiety, psychosomatic complaints, and mood disorders (Sussman 2012). In one study, spouses of workaholic individuals reported marital dissatisfaction, and in another study, children of workaholic individuals were found to be more depressed and parentified (Carroll and Robinson 2000). In Japan, the ill effects of workaholism are recognized, and the term for "death by overwork" is *karoshi*. Companies in Japan are held responsible in wrongful death suits when an individual is overworked to death.

Clinical Case

Jacob is a 45-year-old, white, married financial consultant with no formal psychiatric or medical history. He presents for outpatient therapy at the urging of his wife for being "too distant" from her and their newborn son. Jacob reports that his marriage and family life are "falling apart" because of his overcommitment to work. He states that he has always been a "work-first" type of guy. Throughout his 20s and 30s, he would work up to 100 hours per week, often using large amounts of caffeine on Thursday or Friday nights for a boost of energy to finish the job. During this time, he had no life outside of work, but he describes these years as very satisfying. He was a rising star and frequently received accolades from his boss, who nicknamed him "the machine." He recalls that he did want a family life during this time, but he never had any time to meet anyone. He spent his weekends at home catching up on sleep or doing extra work and always declined offers to socialize. Eventually, his friends from college stopped calling, because they knew he was "married to the job."

Three years ago, Jacob fell in love with his secretary at work, and they were married after a brief romance. He reports that everything was "great" at first. She understood that work was his top priority and seemed content to spend only Sunday evenings together. Over the years, however, she began to express increasing frustration at his inability to disengage from work. Six months ago their first child was born, and she started to "get on him" to spend more time at home and with their son.

Jacob dreads all social obligations that his wife arranges and tells her that he would rather be at home working than socializing. He says yes to every work project out of fear of "letting people down." He finds that he no longer enjoys his work in the same way, but he feels preoccupied by it and constantly thinks about ways to get "back in the game" in order to feel the thrill of being "on top." He wants to succeed in ways he did when he was younger. He constantly seeks approval and yearns for praise from superiors, colleagues, and subordinates. When criticized, he feels anxiety, depressive symptoms, and overwhelming "feelings of failure."

When his wife encourages him to achieve a healthier work-life balance, he lashes out and compares her to "his mother," who regularly "interfered with [his] father's productivity and business ventures." Jacob's father is a hugely successful entrepreneur. Jacob believes that disputes between his parents over work contributed to their separation. Jacob also worries that he will not be as successful as his father.

Jacob states that he would like to spend more time at home, but he feels he cannot cut back on his hours at work. He tried to do so several months ago but found that he could not enjoy life away from the office because all of his thoughts would still be on his work. He then tried to continue to work like before but also spend more time at home. To do this, he increased his caffeine use to "up my energy for everyone," but he ended up becoming irritable, arguing with people both at work and at home. He notes, too, that his wife has recently begun to express concern that he is too tired and distracted to watch his infant son, so she is hesitant to leave the two alone together. He now believes that he is in an "impossible situation." He cannot imagine losing his wife and son, but he also cannot imagine cutting down on his work hours.

In addition to the symptoms already mentioned, Jacob reports insomnia and has had difficulty falling asleep and staying asleep for many years. He has gained about 15 lb in the last 6 months. He reports pain in his lower back and has developed migraine headaches that occur at least once per week. He has never taken a sick day.

Discussion

Effective diagnosis of workaholism is predicated on the identification of its core features, which can be seen in this case study. The term implies excessive amounts of work, but this in itself is not an appropriate measurement. Many external factors may force an individual to work excessively without becoming a workaholic. The original meaning of *workaholism,* as described by Oates (1971), is "the compulsion or the uncontrollable need to work incessantly." This can be delineated as two elements of workaholism: a strong inner drive to work and working excessively hard. This broad definition identifies both the behavioral and cognitive, compulsive elements of workaholism. A third component typically described is degree of work enjoyment, with the typical "classic workaholic" not deriving much enjoyment from his or her work. In this case, Jacob has features of a classic workaholic. Although he started out enjoying his work, his work nature has devolved into excessive work hours, preoccupation and constant compulsion to work, and little enjoyment of work because of work-related stress and inability to manage this stress in productive, healthy ways.

Other, less frequently described, subtypes of workaholics are "work enthusiasts" and "enthusiastic workaholics." Work enthusiasts have high work involvement and enjoyment but low internal/obsessional drive to succeed. Enthusiastic workers exhibit high work involvement and a highly compulsive nature, as well as high levels of work enjoyment.

Currently, workaholism is diagnosed and identified mostly by self-report. Some recent studies have suggested that a simple self-reported identification as workaholic is a key feature (Sussman 2012). To date, there are three validated self-report questionnaires to measure workaholism: the Work Addiction Risk Test (Robinson 1998; Taris et al. 2005), the Workaholism Battery (Andreassen et al. 2011; Spence and Robins 1992), and the Dutch Work Addiction Scale (Shimazu and Schaufeli 2009; Shimazu et al. 2010). At least two other self-report measures have been used: Schedule for Nonadaptive and Adaptive Personality–Workaholism Scale (Clark et al. 1996; McMillan et al. 2002; Woods et al. 2009) and "workaholism behavior measure" (Mudrack and Naughton 2001), although neither is as externally validated. Although these self-report measures diverge in some areas, they all highlight the degree of compulsive involvement with work, time involved with work, and work enjoyment or lack thereof.

Additionally, these reports all identify the carelessness to the interpersonal needs of others inherent in workaholism, such as forgetting important events and neglecting friends and family members (Sussman 2012).

As is seen in Jacob's case, workaholic behavior results in conflict, both internal and external. With Jacob, the responsibilities he had to his family and his own personal health were being overshadowed by his work behaviors. This led to difficulties in his personal life; his wife felt frustrated and angry and even mistrusted his ability to be fully present in order to care for their infant son. Jacob began to feel excessive guilt and inner conflict, and his workaholism ultimately resulted in a severe detriment to his physical and emotional well-being, otherwise known as "burnout" (Sussman 2012). These features are important in making the distinction between healthy excessive enthusiasm in work and work as an addiction. Healthy enthusiasm enriches life; addiction detracts from enjoyment and well-being (Griffiths and Karanika-Murray 2012).

Prevention

Preventing workaholism on the individual level is difficult. Ideally, individual or group therapy could be utilized to address the traits that lead to workaholism, but it may be a challenge to identify such individuals in advance. One could perhaps reach out to children of workaholics or other at-risk individuals, although targeting such a broad group of people may not be feasible in a real-world setting. Preventing workaholism will likely require interventions at more than just the individual level. Societies will need to de-emphasize the value placed on overworking, and organizations will have to employ their various resources (Employee Assistance Programs, periodic work assessments, etc.) to protect workers. More research is needed to identify the types of preventive interventions that would be most effective (Sussman 2012).

Treatment

Treating workaholic individuals can be difficult. Often, the impetus for treatment comes only in the midst of a major crisis such as job loss or the breakup of a relationship. Current literature identifies four barriers to treatment:

1. Unlike substance-related addiction, workaholism cannot be treated with a complete abstinence approach.
2. Community pressure to seek treatment for workaholism is less strong than for substance-related addiction.
3. Workaholism is ego-syntonic, and most patients do not recognize that they have a problem.
4. Workaholics, by definition, have no time to engage in outside endeavors.

Before beginning treatment, practitioners should conduct a full medical and psychiatric workup to rule out any underlying or co-occurring conditions, such as a mood or anxiety disorder. Whereas underlying psychiatric symptoms such as depression and anxiety can be treated with medication, the treatment for workaholism consists of psychotherapeutic engagement with the patient and his or her loved ones.

At the time of this publication, there are no evidence-based interventions for treating work addiction. There are a set of possible strategies for treatment, however. The overall goal in the treatment of work addiction is to achieve a more healthy work-life balance. Thus treatment for work addiction must deal with the underlying causes of addiction and compulsive thoughts. Like other addictions, the most effective treatment for workaholism consists of a multi-prong approach, which may include individual cognitive-behavioral interventions, motivational interviewing, hypnotherapy, family therapy, and group therapy. Additionally, a comprehensive (holistic) approach, including diet modification, exercise, sleep hygiene, relaxation techniques, stress management, assertiveness training, and inclusion of spiritual or existential issues, offers the best hope for recovery. Whereas the majority of interventions are in outpatient settings, inpatient settings may be necessary for individuals on the most severe end of the spectrum.

Cognitive-behavioral therapy interventions specifically address underlying beliefs and attitudes that may cause an individual to overwork. Workaholic individuals should be given the space to explore and potentially mourn early experiences that led them to develop rigid and maladaptive ways of working. Over the course of treatment, the patient should begin to set boundaries between work and home while also scheduling time for self-care, love, and play. During treatment, the he or she should aim to develop greater self-awareness and what Heinz Kohut describes as a "realistic and reliable self-esteem" (Baker and Baker 1987). Other key components of treatment include increasing empathy for others and teaching skills for being more effective at work.

A growing 12-step model initiative, known as Workaholics Anonymous, has gained popularity in recent years. Workaholics Anonymous publishes a book called *The Workaholics Anonymous Book of Recovery* (Workaholics Anonymous World Service Organization 2009a), several pamphlets, the quarterly periodical *Living in Balance*, and a step study guidebook entitled *The Workaholics Anonymous Book of Discovery* (Workaholics Anonymous World Service Organization 2009b). Meetings offer workaholics a safe and supportive environment in which to set goals and to work toward creating a more balanced life with the help of peer support.

Key Points

- Disposition to workaholism includes achievement orientation and desire for higher self-esteem, stressful childhood, competition at work, and feeling more self-efficacious at work than in other settings. Personality traits frequently seen include obsessive compulsion, achievement orientation, perfectionism, and conscientiousness.

- "Classic" workaholism is characterized by excessive work hours, strong obsession with work and compulsion to work while doing other activities, and little enjoyment of the actual work because of the stress, both internal and external, it induces.

- In order to help prevent workaholism, societies will need to de-emphasize the value placed on overworking, and organizations will have to employ their various resources (Employee Assistance Programs, periodic work assessments, etc.) to protect workers.

- There are no evidence-based interventions for workaholism, but cognitive-behavioral therapy–styled therapies, 12-step programs, and other therapies and life changes may be helpful.

References

Andreassen CS, Hetland J, Molde H, Pallesen S: "Workaholism" and potential outcomes in well-being and health in a cross-occupational sample. Stress Health 27:e209–e214, 2011

Baker HS, Baker MN: Heinz Kohut's self psychology: an overview. Am J Psychiatry 144(1):1–9, 1987 3541648

Carroll JJ, Robinson BE: Depression and parentification among adults as related to parental workaholism and alcoholism. Fam J (Alex Va) 8(4):360–367, 2000

Clark LA, Livesley WJ, Schroeder ML, Irish SL: Convergence of two systems for assessing specific traits of personality disorder. Psychol Assess 8(3):294–303, 1996

Griffiths MD: Workaholism: a 21st century addiction. The Psychologist. Bull Br Psychol Soc 24:740–744, 2011

Griffiths MD, Karanika-Murray M: Contextualising over-engagement in work: towards a more global understanding of workaholism as an addiction. J Behav Addict 1(3):87–95, 2012

McMillan LHW, Brady EC, O'Driscoll MP, Marsh NV: A multifaceted validation study of Spence and Robbins' (1992) Workaholism Battery. J Occup Organ Psychol 75(3):357–368, 2002

Mudrack PE, Naughton TJ: The assessment of workaholism as behavioral tendencies: scale development and preliminary empirical testing. Int J Stress Manage 8(2):93–111 2001

Oates WE: Confessions of a Workaholic: The Facts About Work Addiction. New York, World Publishing, 1971

Robinson BE: The workaholic family: a clinical perspective. Am J Fam Ther 26(1):65–75, 1998

Shimazu A, Schaufeli WB: Is workaholism good or bad for employee well-being? The distinctiveness of workaholism and work engagement among Japanese employees Ind Health 47(5):495–502, 2009 19834258

Shimazu A, Schaufeli WB, Taris TW: How does workaholism affect worker health and performance? The mediating role of coping. Int J Behav Med 17(2):154–160, 2010 20169433

Spence JT, Robins AS: Workaholism: definition, measurement, and preliminary results. J Pers Assess 58(1):160–178, 1992 16370875

Sussman S: Workaholism: a review. J Addict Res Ther Suppl 6(1):4120, January 10, 2012

Taris TW, Schaufeli WB, Verhoeven LC: Workaholism in the Netherlands: measurement and implications for job strain and work-nonwork conflict. Appl Psychol 54(1):37–60, 2005

Woods CM, Oltmanns TF, Turkheimer E: Illustration of MIMIC-Model DIF testing with the Schedule for Nonadaptive and Adaptive Personality. J Psychopathol Behav Assess 31(4):320–330, 2009 20442793

Workaholics Anonymous World Service Organization: Workaholics Anonymous Book of Recovery. Menlo Park, CA, Workaholics Anonymous World Services Organization 2009a

Workaholics Anonymous World Service Organization: Workaholics Anonymous Book of Discovery. Menlo Park, CA, Workaholics Anonymous World Services Organization 2009b

Questions

1. What are common barriers that prevent individuals from seeking treatment for workaholism?

   A. Community pressure to seek treatment for workaholism is less strong than for substance-related addiction.
   B. Workaholism is ego-syntonic, and most patients do not recognize that they have a problem.
   C. Workaholics, by definition, have no time to engage in outside endeavors.
   D. Unlike substance-related addiction, workaholism cannot be treated with a complete abstinence approach.
   E. All of the above.

   The correct answer is E.

There are many barriers that prevent individuals from seeking treatment to this oft overlooked condition. All of these options represent examples of such barriers.

2.   What feature of Workaholics Anonymous makes it attractive to some individuals looking for help?

   A. Frequent meetings allowing for peer support when needed.
   B. Addressing underlying cognitive beliefs and attitudes that may cause overwork.
   C. Enhancing motivation to change.
   D. Addressing recurring patterns of behavior that developed in childhood.

The corrected answer is A.

Workaholics Anonymous is a 12-step program that offers workaholic individuals a safe and supportive environment in which to set goals and to work toward creating a more balanced life with the help of peer support. Addressing underlying cognitive beliefs and attitudes that may cause overwork (option B) is a feature of cognitive-behavioral therapy. Enhancing motivation to change (option C) is a feature of motivational interviewing. Addressing recurring patterns of behavior that developed in childhood (option D) is a technique used in psychodynamic psychotherapy.

3.   In addition to working excessively and compulsively, and constant obsession/preoccupation with work, a "classic workaholic" will have what other feature?

   A. Low enjoyment of work.
   B. High enjoyment of work.
   C. A high-end lifestyle that is sustained by work.
   D. No other coexisting behavioral or substance addiction.

The correct answer is A.

The precise definition of a workaholic has not yet been established, although typically many features of a behavioral addiction are seen. However, it is generally agreed that a *classic workaholic* is one who works excessively, feels compelled to work because of inner pressure, and has low enjoyment of work. Frequently, before work becomes an addiction, this individual may derive tremendous enjoyment from

work, but because of the compulsive pursuit and the degree of conflict
this behavior creates, the work becomes detrimental to his or her
health, intimate relationships, and emotional well-being.

4. Irritability, dysphoria, or moodiness experienced when one is forced to
    disengage from work is the characteristic of what core component of a
    behavioral addiction?

    A. Conflict.
    B. Salience.
    C. Withdrawal.
    D. Tolerance.

The correct answer is C.

Workaholism is a true behavioral addiction and has features of the six
core components of addiction (Griffiths and Karanika-Murray 2012).
Withdrawal symptoms may be experienced as irritability, dysphoria, or
moodiness when one is forced to disengage from work. Conflict may be
experienced when the individual is forced to address other demands on
his or her time, such as family. Conflict may be internal, as insight is
gained and a workaholic individual begins to realize that this compulsive
behavior is causing undue distress. Salience occurs when work becomes
the single most important activity in the person's life. This may dominate
the person's thinking and preclude him or her from engaging in other
meaningful activities, because he or she is frequently preoccupied with
work. Tolerance occurs when the amount of hours devoted to work
steadily increases; often one may "chase the buzz" and attempt to replicate the initial pleasure experienced in intense work immersion.

INDEX

Page numbers printed in **boldface** type refer to tables or figures.

Behavioral addictions (*continued*)
  intent and, 12
  marital problems with, 11
  natural history of, 11
  neurotransmitter pathways associated
      with, 17–18
  non-substance behaviors, 4
  pharmacotherapy for, 39–40
  phenomenological characterization
      of, 11
  rewards and, 30
  symptoms of, xiii
  treatment strategies for, 11–12
Behavioral intervention, to diminish
      reward sensitivity, 39
Belviq (lorcaserin), 50
Binge-eating disorder (BED), 45, 47. *See
      also* Food addiction
  treatment of, 39
Bipolar disorder, 33–34, 87–88
Bleuler, Eugen, 177
BMI. *See* Body mass index
Body mass index (BMI), 45
Borderline personality disorder, 165
Bupropion, 50

CASA. *See* Cleptomaniacs and Shoplift-
      ers Anonymous
Case studies
  of attention-deficit/hyperactivity dis-
      order, 105–107
  of E-mail problem use, 103–107
  of exercise, 31–38
  of food addiction, 44–49
  of gambling disorder, 54–58
  of Internet addiction, 82–86
  of Internet gaming disorder, 71–72
  of kleptomania, 115–117
  of love addiction, 161–164
  of obsessive-compulsive disorder,
      104–105
  of sex addiction, 138–140
  of shopping addiction, 175–176
  of substance abuse, 31–38
  of tanning addiction, 188–189

  of texting, 103–107
  of work addiction, 201–203
Catechol O-methyltransferase (COMT),
      128
CBT. *See* Cognitive-behavioral therapy
Chen Internet Addiction Scale, 86
Chinese Internet Addiction Inventory
      (CIAI), **74**
CIAI. *See* Chinese Internet Addiction
      Inventory
CIUS. *See* Compulsive Internet Use
      Scale; Internet Related Problem
      Scale
Clans, **69**
Cleptomaniacs and Shoplifters Anony-
      mous (CASA), 131
Clonazepam, for treatment of klepto-
      mania, 129
Cognitive-behavioral therapy (CBT)
  for treatment of anxiety, 176
  for treatment of disordered exercise,
      39
  for treatment of food addiction, 50
  for treatment of gambling disorder,
      57, 61
  for treatment of Internet addiction, 94
  for treatment of love addiction, 167
  for treatment of sex addiction, 145,
      146
  for treatment of shopping addiction,
      182
  for treatment of work addiction, 204
Community resources, for treatment of
      tanning addiction, 194
Compulsive buying disorder
  criteria for, **181**
  diagnosis of, 180–181
Compulsive Buying Scale, 179–180
Compulsive Internet Use Scale (CIUS),
      74
Compulsive Shoplifters Anonymous
      (CSA), 131
Compulsivity, definition of, 122
COMT. *See* Catechol O-methyltransferase
Console games, **69**